50 Ways to More Calm, Less Stress

SCIENTIFICALLY PROVEN WAYS TO

RELIEVE ANXIETY & BOOST

YOUR MENTAL HEALTH

USING YOUR FIVE SENSES

MEGY KARYDES

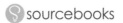

To my loudest cheerleaders and supporters,
Matthew, Chloe & Alex

Published by Sourcebooks
P.O. Box 4410, Naperville, Illinois 60567-4410
(630) 961-3900
sourcebooks.com

Cataloging-in-Publication Data is on file with the Library of Congress.

Printed and bound in China.
OGP 10 9 8 7 6 5 4 3 2 1

CONTENTS

Taste

Smell

Hear

See

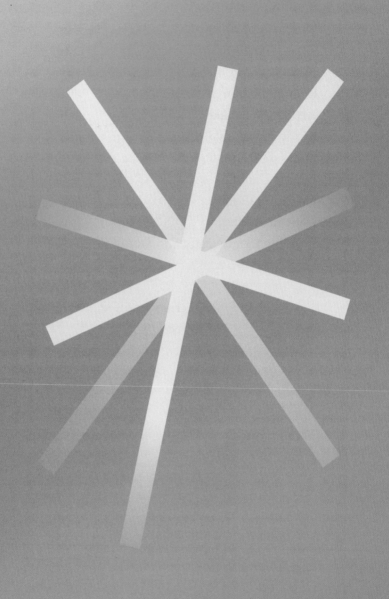

INTRODUCTION

Most experts will tell you that if you're feeling over-whelmed, try taking some deep breaths. Or do yoga. This is all fine and good if you love to meditate or do a daily yoga practice. For some of us, these activities don't work. At least not immediately.

Many of us are busier than we've ever been. Even before COVID-19 wreaked havoc on our lives, we were expected to be tethered to our digital devices and responsive twenty-four seven. Kids need our attention. Elderly parents need care-giving. We have households to upkeep. Dinner to prepare. Doctor appointments to make. No wonder our brains are on fire and can't seem to rest. And now you want me to add a daily yoga practice? Are you out of your mind?

I started to realize I was having a hard time "relaxing" my brain just before I left my corporate job as a marketing director. I couldn't turn off work no matter how hard I tried. I finally resigned so I could start my own marketing and communications agency, which allowed me to choose whom I work with and to take on as much—or as little—work as I wanted.

Now on my own, I have more control of my life, which is true, but that doesn't mean I'm not stressed. The stress just shifted. Now it's all about my clients and meeting my editors' deadlines while still attending to my personal life. I want to make sure my kids are getting a good education while being physically and mentally stimulated with extracurricular activities. I also want to ensure we're eating healthy diets at home while still supporting our community by eating out and shopping locally—not to mention staying physically fit by exercising and mentally fit by attending cultural events.

That same stress buildup was happening in my head: no matter how hard I tried to do breathing exercises or yoga to calm my brain and allow my body the opportunity to relax, I was on overdrive. My brain felt like my computer screen with thirty-five tabs open, and I was unable to decide which one was most important and needed my focus.

During a media interview for a client, I arranged for a radio host to participate in forest therapy at the Morton Arboretum in Lisle, Illinois. According to the Association of Nature and Forest Therapy Guides and Programs, *forest therapy*, also known as *shinrin-yoku*, refers to the practice of spending time in forested areas for the purpose of enhancing health, wellness, and happiness. The practice follows the general principle that it is beneficial to spend time bathing in the atmosphere of the forest.

When in the forest, something clicked for me. Sitting still and meditating didn't work for me. My mind kept racing. Yoga didn't work for me. My mind was stressing out trying to get the poses right so I didn't embarrass myself by falling. But taking a walk in the woods, forcing myself to try and identify the farthest sound, then listen to the closest one, hear the rustling happening beneath my feet with every step, inhale the fresh air, or squint my eyes from the sun's rays sneaking through the tree branches did something for me. I couldn't remember the last time I felt so much peace and calm. It felt magical. I realized there were other ways I could calm my mind. By taking the time to explore my senses, I could stop just long enough to appreciate what was happening in my life at that moment.

By then, I'd already been writing in my journal every morning. During that sunny afternoon in the woods, I felt something similar to my morning writing practice, which also forced me to be still and appreciate the tactile feeling of writing something down but also cleared my head through a cleansing brain dump. Different experiences and yet similar feelings.

What other calming experiences have we neglected because we never bothered to appreciate what each of our five senses affords us on a daily basis?

Don't get me wrong, a daily meditation or yoga practice can do wonders for many people. As can traditional therapy. But like anything in life, there is no one-size-fits-all approach to finding what calms us because we're all so uniquely different in our circumstances, our lives, our finances, and our interests.

In fact, not being able to sit still and meditate or be alone with our thoughts for extended periods of time isn't that unusual. In a series of eleven studies, psychologist Timothy Wilson and his colleagues at University of Virginia and Harvard found that many people did not enjoy spending even short bursts of time alone in a room with nothing to do but think, ponder, or daydream—to the point that they'd rather inflict pain on themselves.

"The mind is designed to engage with the world," Wilson said in an article published in *UVA Today*. "Even when we are by ourselves, our focus usually is on the outside world. And without training in meditation or thought-control techniques, which still are difficult, most people would prefer to engage in external activities."

This book is for those people—for those of you who want to invite more serenity into your lives and are willing to explore different ways to embrace it.

Emboldened by my feelings in the forest, I decided to explore different ways each of our five senses can help contribute to bringing more calm and less stress into our lives. Whether the activity involves touch, sight, taste, smell, or sound, each one includes research or science-backed studies that explain why it offers health and wellness benefits as well as ways you can try to incorporate it into your life.

Try one. Try them all. Before you dismiss one as "not for you" though, why not give it a go? If nothing else, you can confirm it's not a good fit for you. Or you may just find yourself with a brand-new interest that you love.

It's important to note that what works for you today might not work for you tomorrow, next month, or next year.

Just like each of our circumstances is different, our circumstances change. A parent might suddenly need help on a daily basis, or their job has changed and requires more travel. Try something new, and see if that might work for your current circumstances.

This book is for those who want—who need—more calm and less stress in their lives. It's for those who want to quiet the noise in their heads long enough so they can think about what matters most to them. It's for those who want to start or return to a creative practice. It's for those who want to spend more time with the people they love. It's for busy parents who don't feel like they have even ten minutes to unwind before they drop into bed, exhausted, every night. It's for college students who are trying to cram in quality study time between working a part-time job and juggling an internship. It's for caregivers who have to care for their elderly parents and are ready to tear their hair out because they're not equipped to deal with the stress.

If you picked up this book and read this far, this book is for you. It's for us.

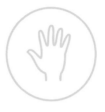

Touch

If you truly get in touch with a piece of carrot, you get in touch with the soil, the rain, the sunshine. You get in touch with Mother Earth and eating in such a way, you feel in touch with true life, your roots, and that is meditation. If we chew every morsel of our food in that way we become grateful and when you are grateful, you are happy.

THICH NHAT HANH

(1)

The Magic of Gardening

There are few things that taste better than your own homegrown tomato. Picking that first ripe tomato off the vine during the height of summer feels like a special treat.

"When you're in the garden, it seduces you," Ron Finley, a Los Angeles–based community activist and self-proclaimed "Gangster Gardener" said as part of his MasterClass introduction. "There is magic in creating something with your own hands. Growing your own food gives you power. Once you have it, it's something that can never be taken away from you."

The enthusiasm for gardening has grown, especially since the start of the COVID-19 pandemic in 2020. According to Minneapolis-based firm Axiom Marketing, many homeowners said they began gardening because it gave them something to do while stuck at home, provided a source of exercise, and helped to cope with stress. I count myself among those who began gardening in earnest in 2020. While my mother has been a gardener her whole life, and I lived in a home with a backyard for twenty years, I was never motivated to take advantage of gardening until I found myself with extra time and wanted to be somewhat productive with it.

I stumbled across a neighborhood group sharing free seeds, so I walked there and picked up half a dozen packets, which included tomato and pepper seeds. Within a few days, one upcycled feta cheese plastic container, two red plastic cups, and three metal cans were lined up along my west-facing windowsill, filled with soil I scooped up from my backyard. I dropped in a few white cherry, black cherry, and yellow pear tomato seeds. Almost two weeks later, my first sprouts began to appear, and I cried. Never having grown anything from seed, I was amazed and so happy. I immediately told the woman who shared her seeds with me. Her response? "Aren't seeds just f*cking magic?"

I babied those tiny (we're talking half an inch here) seedlings and checked on them religiously every morning to make sure they didn't die. I was convinced they weren't going to make it. I watered them, I talked to them, I made sure they were getting enough sunlight. Once our Chicago weather permitted, my mom came and helped me gently place my babies in the soil. Feeling the cool soil in my hands felt powerful. That summer, I grew my first tomatoes from seed, and the taste was unimaginable. I was hooked.

I'm not alone. While 2020 might have encouraged many people to start gardening, their enthusiasm, like mine, didn't wane. Axiom Marketing's research showed 92 percent of surveyed home gardeners spent the same or more time and money on gardening activities in 2021, and 20 percent of those respondents said that gardening lowers their stress level, which is one of the reasons they garden.

Research shows that direct contact with natural environments results in important positive health outcomes, which we'll see in a number of the activities mentioned throughout this book. "Engagement with both wild and cultivated natural places improves self-esteem and mood, reduces stress and anxiety and fosters mental well-being," the research noted.

Another reason playing in the dirt might be good for our mental health? *Mycobacterium vaccae*, a soil-derived bacterium with immunoregulatory and stress resilience properties.

Yes, bacteria can help our mental health. Stay with me.

Previous studies have shown that *Mycobacterium vaccae* increases serotonin in the prefrontal cortex, which modulates anxiety. While working as a research fellow at the University of Bristol, lead author Dr. Christopher Lowry and a team of scientists published research in the journal *Neuroscience* that suggested a type of friendly bacteria found in soil may affect the brain in a similar way to antidepressants.

Shawna Coronado is a wellness and lifestyle authority and author of several books. She's been advocating time spent in the garden for years, and one of the main reasons she loves getting her hands dirty is because of the benefits of *Mycobacterium vaccae*.

"While we know that the bacterium strain *Mycobacterium vaccae* has been shown to trigger the release of serotonin when a person has direct skin-to-soil contact, there is also further proof that dopamine levels increase in the brain when we participate in green activities," Coronado wrote in her book *The Wellness Garden: Grow, Eat, and Walk Your Way to Better Health.*

"Both serotonin and dopamine are pleasure-center neurotransmitters that are associated with happiness, pleasure, and love," Coronado added.

TRY IT

1. You don't need a huge backyard to reap the benefits of gardening. You simply need sunlight and some outdoor space. You can even place a small container along a small terrace if that's the only space you have or on a windowsill if you have no space at all, as long as the area gets a decent amount of sunlight throughout the day. Before you invest in any containers or plants to grow, find the area that offers the most sunlight. Will you be growing in a container garden, your backyard, or on a rooftop? Consider your environment as many plants will require direct sunlight to grow.

2. Once you have identified your area, figure out your climate zone so you can grow plants that will thrive in your climate. Plug your zip code in the USDA plant hardiness zone map (planthardiness.ars.usda.gov), and once you know your hardiness zone, identify the fruits, vegetables, flowers, and herbs that you can grow in your environment.

3 Next up: Do you want to grow flowers, vegetables, fruits, herbs, or a combination? Do you want to be able to cut flowers or grow vegetables to eat during the summer or year-round? Don't forget, gardening is an experiment. You can always change things up the next year based on what happens this year.

4 While you don't need a lot of gardening tools to get the job done, you will need a few. It's smart to invest in good tools, so they'll last. Don't forget your local "Buy Nothing" or "Free Box" groups. Many people offer up their garden tools for free when they find they have too many, no longer use them, or are moving. Here are some items to consider adding to your gardening tool kit, based on what you're growing:

- A hand trowel or scooper to fill pots and planters
- A hand rake and weeder to loosen soil and remove weeds in a garden, respectively
- A pruner to make clean cuts of stems
- Gardening gloves to protect your hands and keep them clean
- A garden hoe to remove grass and weeds while also making space to add seeds and bulbs in the ground
- If you're going to be on your knees a lot, a padded kneeler or portable seat to save your knees and back
- If you're going to be transporting a lot of soil around your garden, a wheelbarrow
- A watering can or garden hose (or both, depending on where you're gardening)
- Wide-brim sun hat and garden clogs or boots

* If you're planting vegetables, signage labels so you know where and what you planted

* **BONUS:** A hori hori knife. I didn't know what this was until someone gifted it to me, and I wish I had known about it sooner as it's great for slicing through roots and other coarse garden tasks, and many come with measurements etched into one side of the blade to help with planting.

5. If you're planning to grow vegetables or fruits, you may want to test your soil in advance. Your local cooperative extension office can test your soil sample for pH and nutrient levels (some states charge a nominal fee for the service). The soil analysis usually takes a few weeks to process, and your results may include suggested amendments specific to your region.

6. Decide whether you're going to grow from seeds or transplant seedlings. If you're going to start from seed, figure out when you need to start them indoors (based on the last expected frost date) so they'll be ready to transplant outdoors when the weather conditions allow.

7. Prepare your garden bed by pulling out any weeds or clearing any existing vegetation. It's important to remove as much of the weeds as possible because you don't want your new plants to be competing for nutrients with weeds. Add a thick layer of compost (either your own or purchased).

8. Once you're ready to plant, take great care to transplant your seedlings into the soil. Be mindful of how deep in the soil the seedlings should be planted and how far apart they should be

spaced. This information is usually on the label of purchased plants, or you can find information online. This is also where a tool like the hori hori can come in handy with its measurements etched on the side of the blade.

9 Water well and mulch liberally.

10 Keep up with maintenance and enjoy your garden throughout the season.

2

Write It Out

Julia Cameron might very well be the doyenne of jour-naling as a form of meditation. Since its publication, her book *The Artist's Way* has sold more than four million copies and inspires readers to embark on their own creative journey to find their purpose through the simple yet power-ful daily practice called Morning Pages. She calls on readers to dispense with their digital devices and put pen to paper to write three pages of longhand, stream of consciousness writing. She's adamant about the practice: three pages every morning without fail. For most people, this exercise takes about thirty to forty minutes.

Night owls aren't out of luck. Go ahead and write in the evenings if that's better for you, but the spirit of Morning Pages is designed to help you clear your mind and prepare you for the day ahead, hence the reason for doing them in the morning.

Like many of the activities I share throughout the book, I was dubious about this one, and I *am* a writer. In the spirit of giving it a shot, I started writing my Morning Pages almost a decade ago and haven't stopped since. Why? Because it works for me. What initially began as clumsy and cumbersome and feeling like a chore now feels calming and cathartic. I look forward to grabbing a favorite pen, sitting with my beautiful journal and hot cup of coffee, no matter the season, to write those Morning Pages religiously.

For those who just don't love the idea of writing longhand, are self-conscious of their handwriting, or want some added motivation or accountability, 750words.com allows you to type your Morning Pages and keep track of how many words you've written. Unlike a blog page, what you write is completely private—no one will see it except you. No one will grade your grammar. No one will judge you.

The site cheers you on and tries to motivate you to write those 750 words (which is equivalent to about three longhand Morning Pages). When you sign up, the first email you receive encourages you to write three days in a row in order to receive your first badge (a Turkey badge). If you write consecutively for five days, you score the Penguin badge. The site offers monthly challenges to keep you motivated and feel part of a larger community. It is free to try for the first month and then five dollars a month to continue.

Scientific studies support the notion that journaling has a host of benefits, from helping with memory and communications skills to better sleep, a stronger immune system, and improved self-confidence. Dr. James W. Pennebaker agrees.

Pennebaker is a social psychologist at the University of Texas at Austin and considered the pioneer of writing therapy. He focuses on how to use writing to help recover from traumatic or disturbing events and is also the author of several books on the mind-body benefits of journaling, including *Opening Up by Writing It Down: How Expressive Writing Improves Health and Eases Emotional Pain.*

According to Pennebaker, labeling emotions and acknowledging traumatic events—both natural outcomes of journaling—have a known positive effect on people and are often incorporated into traditional talk therapy. Some of those positive effects, fairly generalized, include less ruminating about problems, better sleeping, and improvements in health and social functioning.

While the tactile experience of journaling doesn't have to be focused on traumatic events, a study published in the American Psychological Association's *Journal of Experimental Psychology: General* indicates that expressive writing reduces intrusive and avoidant thoughts about negative events and improves working memory. "These improvements, researchers believe, may in turn free up our cognitive resources for other mental activities, including our ability to cope more effectively with stress," wrote Siri Carpenter in her article for the association's website, "A New Reason for Keeping a Diary."

The study's results suggest "that at least for fairly minor life problems, something as simple as writing about the problem for 20 minutes can yield important effects not only in terms of physical health and mental health, but also in terms of cognitive abilities," said Adriel Boals, coauthor of the study.

Pennebaker agrees that keeping a journal helps us process things and organize what's happening in our minds—even for those of us who may not be using it to process traumatic experiences. By putting pen to paper, our working memory improves, since our brains are freed from the enormously taxing job of processing different types of experiences, and we can then sleep better at night. This in turn improves our immune systems and our moods; we go to work feeling refreshed, perform better, and socialize more. Pennebaker adds there's no single magic moment, but you know it works. "One important sign is that you may go minutes, even hours without thinking about the event that you were obsessing about every minute in the days before writing," he explained. "And, over time, your thoughts about the upsetting event become less present and, when they do occur, less troubling."

—————————————— TRY IT ——————————————

1 You don't need a fancy journal and pen to get started, but I love my pens and journals, so I usually buy pens that write smoothly and journals with a great cover design. It feels like a treat to me to sit down every morning and feel the pen and journal in my hands before taking a deep breath and starting to write.

2 Pennebaker recommends we find a spot where we won't be disturbed and start writing. "You are writing for yourself

and no one else," he told me. "If you can't think what to write about, just start writing about how you are feeling or what you are seeing or why you are writing in the first place. Promise you will write for at least 10 minutes and, if you want, you can tear up what you've written. If you run out of things to say, repeat what you have already written."

3. In some cases, people think, "I don't want to write about this upsetting event because it will just upset me further." In those cases, Pennebaker said, the problem is you're already thinking about it all the time. "Once you start writing, if you feel as though you are getting too upset, stop!" At this point, perhaps it's better to write about something else.

4. What to write if something doesn't come naturally to you? Think of something that's on your mind, something you've been enjoying lately, or something you're excited to try. Remember, your writing isn't going to be read by anyone. It's not *meant* to be read by anyone. It's not going to be edited for grammar, so don't worry about how it reads or if the words are spelled correctly. It's just for you.

5. If it's still too hard to think of something to write, there are a number of places where you can get writing prompts sent to you daily. Cameron also wrote *The Right to Write*, which includes a writing exercise at the end of each chapter, such as asking readers to describe a situation that is consuming their thoughts, like getting used to a new boss or living with a partner. Anything can be a topic you can write about, and she

encourages readers to "write about things you would like to see more clearly."

6 Consider this experience an experiment, and plan to write a minimum of ten minutes a day for three consecutive days. If, at the end, you are not feeling better, maybe writing is not for you. But here's the thing: if you want to write for more than three days, do it. "Most people find that writing just three or four days is all they need sometimes," Pennebaker said. Remember, you are the judge about what is helpful for you, and each of us has to find our own path. There is no one right or true way of writing.

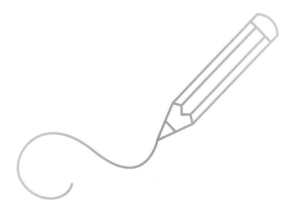

3

Lose Yourself in a Doodle

When we're bored or want to pass the time, we might grab a pen and start to doodle or sketch. In the past, teachers would scold students for doodling during class because they thought students weren't paying attention. Yet research shows that doodling isn't done as a form of distraction and, in fact, might help those who want to focus.

Even twenty-six former American presidents doodled. Theodore Roosevelt drew animals and children, Ronald Reagan drew cowboys and football players, and John F. Kennedy drew dominoes. In his book *Presidential Doodles: Two Centuries of Scribbles, Scratches, Squiggles, and Scrawls from the Oval Office*, historian David Greenberg wrote, "Soon after Somali militiamen killed eighteen American soldiers in Mogadishu on October 3, 1993, President Clinton convened his national security team in the White House. As recalled by the counterterrorism expert Richard Clarke, the president sat silently as his aides reviewed the situation. Then, Clarke wrote, 'When they had talked themselves out, Clinton stopped doodling and looked up. "Okay, here's what we're going to do."'"

According to Clarke, Clinton could afford to doodle because he already knew what had to be done. Or could it be that the act of doodling helped unlock part of his brain so he could figure out what needed to be done?

Dana DuMont is an artist and educator who teaches a meditative botanical drawing class she designed for Lewis Ginter Botanical Garden in Richmond, Virginia. Participants in her class love natural spaces and gardens, and she noticed many of them are willing to experiment with drawing and painting materials as a way to add more creative and calming time to their days.

One of DuMont's students was Liz Hambrick, who was drawn to her class because it sounded like an accessible route to meditation. Hambrick admits she's never had success with more traditional types of meditation but she's a doodler by nature and knows how relaxing it can be not to have to try to produce something particular and to let things flow.

At one point in her life, she found herself suffering from a lack of focus and concentration (more than usual). She was hoping for a new lease on life following hip replacement surgeries, but instead of getting better, the active, athletic, and outdoorsy person who loved walking long distances felt robbed. She had the energy and desire but no longer the physical ability.

"I became extremely depressed, something that took several years to overcome, until I could reinvent and accept a new me," Hambrick said. "Fortunately, I have always been visually creative, and I still had the capability intact to pursue that side of myself. Depression, however, is the thief of creativity, so I had to get out from under that before I could enjoy that side of life."

To help manage her condition, Hambrick did everything from kayaking and joining a drum circle to journaling and knitting, but none of those activities gives her the same type of healing, undemanding, and meditative experience that drawing and painting give her.

"I can become completely lost and focused when I draw and paint, and the thinking part of my brain automatically becomes still and quiet," Hambrick told me. "I have a profound love of nature, it always heals me, and all my artwork is inspired by being immersed in it."

When she learned of DuMont's class, the short online format of the Lewis Ginter Botanical Garden class appealed to her, so she signed up. The experience turned out to be exactly what she needed and was almost therapeutic.

"It was like somebody shoved me over a threshold without me even knowing it," she said. The threshold was a gateway to another world where she could find peace and just be, spending time with herself and a pen and paper. "It got me through the worst of times," she explained. Since the class began, she has continued to practice her healing art of drawing nearly daily. "It's something I find myself needing to do. If I don't do it for a few days, I get twitchy."

DuMont isn't surprised by Hambrick's response to the class. "The experience is all about releasing stress, finding center, and creating an additional instrument to carry along in our balancing gear," DuMont told me.

One of the reasons DuMont chooses to focus on flowers and botanicals in her class is she feels they elicit a sense of hope and pleasure. "Drawing from observation while adding repetitive design elements and playful embellishment allows the mind to wander, and because individuals seek out ways to express their own visions of contentment, beauty, peace, perspective and the like, I combined these ideas," she added.

Doodling can be just as helpful to calm the body and mind, and DuMont calls doodling a brilliant way to engage your senses without tuning out. "Many of us can't be present or attentive in meetings, classes, etc. without doing it," she said. "It allows some of us to listen and process ideas more fully or to let thoughts find a place to rest."

Fear of Failure

While doodling or sketching can be calming, some people may feel nervous because they're novices or they won't be as good as they'd like to be. "The very act of taking an art class is a risk-taking experience on some level," DuMont said. "People might be interested in drawing but are unsure of how to use some of the materials, what to bring along, or how comfortable they'll feel creating work in a public space."

For some, taking a class online allows them to go at their own pace without feeling judged by an instructor or other classmates, and that's totally fine. Online classes can also feel a bit safer since you can turn off the camera and not be visible.

Still, many participants enjoy the experience of taking this type of class in person, according to DuMont, because they want to share their work and ideas as they relax and get into the flow. "The sharing—in any space—adds another level of community, creative brainstorming, and connection," she noted. "And yes, laughter, kindness and openness to experimentation organically grow so that, by the end of each class, people leave lighter and more energized."

—————————— TRY IT ——————————

1. If you'd like to experiment with doodling or sketching, no special skills are required. Just grab a pen and some paper (heck, you can even doodle on napkins!), and let your hand and mind wander. Enjoy the tactile experience of holding a writing instrument and letting it glide along the surface.

2. Invest in a writing instrument or paper that allows your hand to almost effortlessly dance along the paper. Some markers glide softly along silky papers, for example. Or buy a felt-tip pen and small notebook to have on hand, and pull both out when you just want a little doodling break.

3. If you don't know where to begin, repetitive geometric shapes created around a base of a circle can give you some initial direction. Then let your hand continue to see what you come up with.

4 There are hundreds of online doodling or sketching classes that you can sign up for, and like DuMont noted, you can keep your camera turned off if you're not comfortable being visible if it's a live class. Or watch a video online, and follow along at your own pace.

5 Finally, there's always the option of taking an in-person class. Check out local art schools, libraries, botanic gardens, and community centers or community colleges. Ask friends and neighbors for recommendations. You never know who might be interested in taking a class with you!

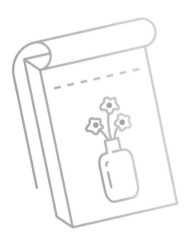

Painting for Perspective

It's no surprise that when our minds wander, it's often to the territory of unpleasant thoughts. We may find ourselves worrying about our health, our kids, our parents, our jobs, wars, or finances. Engaging in mindfulness practices helps us stay present in the current moment, and research has shown that people are happier if they are paying attention to the present moment, even if what they are doing is an unpleasant task.

Some, like Michele Weldon, are finding that creating art is a form of respite and escape from their daily worries. Weldon, now in her midsixties, returned to creating art after a twenty-four-year hiatus. She leads a rather public life and one that is often intensely scrutinized. She's worked as a journalist for more than forty years for major global media outlets and is the author of six nonfiction books, including her most recent, *Act Like You're Having a Good Time: Essays.*

But for Weldon, creating art is for no one's enjoyment or benefit but her own. "I feel free," Weldon said.

Weldon experiments with colors and techniques, switching mediums from pastels to charcoal to oil paints. It allows her to see things differently, she said. "I notice shadows on a desk differently, sunlight through clouds differently, the colors of a bird's wing. It allows me to be mindful and to develop clarity without expectation or reward."

The benefit of creating art doesn't end with how Weldon feels. It extends to her body as well.

"It soothes my mind and also my body as the tight specificity of a paint brush stroke or a single line from a pastel stick can make a huge difference," she added. "Precision is required. I can also use larger strokes that are liberating and surprising."

One doesn't need formal experience to create art.

In 2009, *I Remember Better When I Paint*, a documentary about the impact of nonpharmaceutical approaches on persons affected by Alzheimer's disease and related disorders, aired on public television stations throughout the country. Through interviews with renowned neurologists, caregivers, and family members affected by these diseases, the film shared *why art works* in terms of the brain's hard wiring.

In a review of the film, Rick J. Scheidt, PhD, shared some of the highlights. "Dr. Sam Gandy of Mount Sinai Hospital notes that the parietal lobe, stimulated through creative activities such as art and music, is unaffected by AD until its later phases," Scheidt wrote. "Dr. Avertano Noronha of University of Chicago informs us that emotional communication is possible for those with AD [Alzheimer's disease] because the amygdala, linked to emotional reactivity, apparently remains intact. (The neighboring hippocampus, responsible for short-term memory processes, suffers damage early in the disease.)"

Art therapists explain it in a slightly different way. "When they are given paints, markers, any kind of media for art making and their hands are involved, and their muscles are involved, things are tapped in them that are genuine, and active, and alive that don't get tapped in our normal day social interaction…so the creative arts *bypass the limitations* and they simply go to the strengths," Judy Holstein, former director of adult day services at CJE SeniorLife in Chicago, said.

The benefits of making art aren't limited to those with Alzheimer's disease or dementia. The activity helps us to communicate using our hands and vision. It gives us permission to create and focus on what we're creating as opposed to everything else going on around us.

"Like mindfulness, the most well documented benefit of art is also decreased negative affect," Lydia Fogo wrote in her thesis published in the *University of Tennessee at Chattanooga Scholar*.

Creating art, whether it's drawing or painting, can relieve stress, anxiety, and depression. It can help with expressive communication and prevent or minimize cognitive decline. And one is never too old to start (or start again).

Weldon always loved being creative and drew, painted, and sketched as a child. Her parents encouraged her and would hang up her acrylic paintings in hallways and bathrooms of their house. She took art classes in high school and college and continued to paint into her twenties. She stopped when her children were born, as she simply couldn't fit it in.

It was only after her youngest went away to college in 2012 that she finally had weekends off, and she was desperate to get back to her creative self, so she enrolled in adult classes at the Art Institute of Chicago. Later, she took virtual pastel drawing classes through the Ninety-Second Street Y every Saturday throughout the year.

Her time is still crunched these days with an intense work schedule, even working remotely, so she sketches or paints at home in the breakfast room, with an easel or drawing board where the light is good.

Weldon made friends with two others she met in 2012 at the Art Institute while taking classes, and they now meet on Saturdays at each other's homes to sketch, draw, and paint for a few hours. "It is an added plus if you can do this with like-minded friends," she said. "I cannot imagine life without their friendships."

TRY IT
---

1. Remember, creating art should be enjoyable, not stressful, and it helps to think about creating for yourself and no one else. Weldon does create some pieces, frames them, and hangs them up in her home or gives them as gifts, but that's not the point and certainly not the end goal. "Do it for

yourself, not for accolades or approval," she recommends. "It is rewarding to have compliments on your work, but do not endeavor to create art so that others will like it."

2 If you're unsure of what to tackle, take some time to enjoy a field trip to an art museum. Let yourself take in the beauty of the artwork and see what you're drawn to. You may think you don't like watercolors but then find yourself appreciating how the colors blend into each other. Or maybe you already like acrylic paintings but didn't realize it's because you really enjoy seeing the details in the brushstrokes.

3 Invest in a few pieces including a canvas, pencils, colored pencils, markers and pens, or brushes and paint. No need to invest in a whole arts supply store—just a few basics will do for now. The point is to get started with a few things and enjoy the process.

4 There are a number of art classes offered at local colleges, community centers, and art schools if you prefer guided instruction. Or check out tutorial videos on YouTube to get started with a few basics.

5 Finally, remember to be kind to yourself. Even if your work isn't frame-worthy, there is beauty in the process. Consider how your body feels as you're working on a piece—from thinking about what you're doing to feeling the paintbrush in your hand gliding over the canvas or paper. Let your mind be present with your activity. While Weldon does frame some

of her pieces, she's not shy in admitting that she hides a lot of her work because she made mistakes or doesn't like how a piece turned out. But she never berates herself. Instead, she tells herself next week is another chance to build something of beauty with her bare hands.

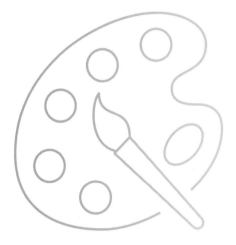

5

Move Your Body

Most of us know sitting for long periods of time can be detrimental to our health and well-being. One study noted prolonged sitting (which usually occurs in front of a television set or computer or while driving) leads to substantially greater health risks than had been previously reported. On average, 60 percent of waking hours of adults is spent being sedentary, and sedentary behavior, such as sitting in front of a television, is linked to obesity, diabetes, impaired glucose uptake, and insulin resistance, all of which lead to higher medical costs and poorer quality of life. Perhaps surprising to some, especially those who still get a workout in during the day, is those who are more active throughout the day and sit less are better off than those who exercise once per day and spend the rest of the day being sedentary.

Erica Hornthal is a board-certified dance/movement

therapist and licensed clinical professional counselor. She's also founder and CEO of Chicago Dance Therapy and author of *Body Aware*, a guidebook that addresses how the way we move impacts who we are.

Movement, including dance, is not about exercising or even knowing how to dance, according to Hornthal. Instead, she encourages us to recognize our relationship to movement, explore our current movement habits, and expand our own range of and capacity for movement so we can improve our mental health and create a life full of meaning and purpose.

"When we move more, we feel more," Hornthal said. "And sometimes that's feeling better. But sometimes it's just feeling, period."

Dance isn't just an art form. Hornthal reminds us it's one of our first forms of communication. Before we could learn how to speak as babies, even before we learned to walk, we were dancing to communicate our needs. "So if we look at dance as more of a way to communicate and not just as an aesthetic or a skill or an art, then we start to uncover why dance is so important," she said.

Unlike taking a dance class or learning a certain style of dance, dance as movement is looking at how we connect to rhythm, how we connect to our bodies, and how we express ourselves beyond words.

We could be trying everything possible to change our mindset, but without being aware of how we're showing up in our bodies, we won't appreciate the benefits since what's happening with our bodies contributes to what's happening in our minds. "If our body isn't changing at all, it's like pulling a weed but leaving the root," Hornthal said.

Most of us are very aware of mental fatigue and burnout in an emotional sense, but we may not immediately recognize how it shows up in our bodies until we feel a physical ache or pain. Hornthal recommends reconnecting people to movement by incorporating it into what's happening to them on a daily basis. Instead of asking ourselves how we are doing or feeling, Hornthal encourages us to ask how we are *moving*.

Let's say you're sitting on the couch; she'll press you to consider what parts of you are moving right now. You might notice your breathing or that you can feel your heart beating. You might swallow or blink. Involuntary movements are happening all the time, and you begin to notice them. Once clients start to notice there is movement already happening throughout their day and they don't have to intentionally schedule something like yoga or go to the gym, they start to find other ways to incorporate and increase movement.

"Then at some point, there's kind of a switch that gets flipped," Hornthal said. "It's like they notice they have so much potential for movement. They'll move their arm in a way they've never moved, and before you know it, it kind of looks like dance."

Hornthal added this movement is literally letting your body speak its native language as opposed to teaching it.

The power of dance is that it also incorporates all the senses. Starting from the top of your body, we're taking in air and we're breathing, which gives us the opportunity for sense of scent and even taste. We're touching things as we move. We can either listen to music or not and keep our eyes open or closed.

"I think that's what makes dance such a healing experience," Hornthal noted. "It gives us the opportunity to tap into so many senses that we don't even take advantage of."

She admits she's biased because she's a dancer and loves to use movement, but she reminds us that anytime we incorporate the arts into our life, it's undoubtedly going to help us increase the use of our senses and the awareness of our senses. "And when we're in our senses, we're in the moment," she said. "We can't be worried about the future. We can't be scared about the past. We have no choice but to be in our bodies when we are aware of our senses."

TRY IT

For those interested in adding more movement to their day, Hornthal shared a few ways to get started.

1. Start by noticing what you're feeling in your body. Bring your attention to how different parts of your body feel. Are your shoulders tense? Are they up around your ears instead of relaxed? You might make the connection with how your body feels and how this impacts your mental health. "For me, when my shoulders are tight, I'm already stressed," Hornthal said. Then you start to think of ways to improve your situation, because if your body and mind are stressed, they're not going to improve unless the situation changes.

2. If your shoulders are tight because you're stressed, and it's going to impact your mental health, you can ask yourself what you can do to lessen the tension. "I can start to roll my shoulders, I can squeeze my shoulders and then try to let them go, I can massage my shoulders or ask someone [I] know or a loved one to massage them for me," Hornthal recommended. "It's more movement than anything else. But if you think about it, a lot of those movements are dance warm-ups."

3. Keep thinking about how you're moving right now. If something's not working well or not feeling right, give yourself permission to move in another way. Get out of a chair, move to the bed, loosen the grip on your steering wheel as you're driving. None of these things are a piece of choreography, but they are all movement, which is the core component of dance.

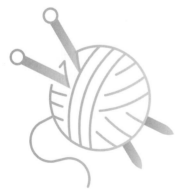

(6)

In the Loop

When Melissa Blount, PhD, took up embroidery as part of a project to memorialize Black women and girls killed by violence in Chicago, she admitted she only knew one stitch. "And I don't even think I was doing that stitch correctly," she said, laughing.

Doing something with her hands and creating a community circle to come together and embroider was what she needed to help her get through some difficult times.

It's also what she recommends to clients.

Blount is a licensed clinical psychologist. One of the reasons she recommends the practice of needlework, whether it takes the form of cross-stitching, embroidery, knitting, crocheting, quilting, or something else, is that it works in the same way meditation does.

"It dampens that cortisol fight-or-flight response that

we all find ourselves in," Blount said. "But any activity that engages every part of yourself and your consciousness is going to promote a relaxing response from your body versus a hypervigilant, 'I need to be aware of all threats and dangers' response. It really is a full body experience."

For others, like Shannon Downey, embroidery is a different kind of therapeutic exercise. By all accounts, Downey was leading a successful life as the founder and owner of a busy digital marketing company in Chicago. What clients and participants weren't seeing was she was working around the clock, constantly connected to her digital devices, and feeling burned out, empty, and exhausted. There was no creativity left in the tank, and she felt she wasn't doing her best work because she was stuck on autopilot.

"I hated everything," Downey admitted. "I felt like I needed some digital-analog balance in my life."

As a self-proclaimed *Star Trek* superfan, she came across a *Star Trek* cross-stitch pattern. Having learned how to stitch in fifth grade, she thought this was something fun she could try.

"I bought this pattern and I stitched Captain Picard that weekend," she said. "And I was like, 'Oh my God, this is revolutionary.' Immediately, I knew that this was exactly what I needed. So I started stitching every day."

Like Blount shared, one of the reasons Downey quickly took to this type of embroidery is it involves her hands, touch, and movement.

"You're using your hands in such a way that it almost mirrors how you use a device," Downey explained.

To be fair, she tried to meditate in the traditional sense of sitting still, being quiet, and breathing. It just didn't work for her. "I'm really antsy. And I'm antsy because I'm so used to having a device in my hand," Downey added. She likened the experience to feeling like she was missing a body part.

"When you're stitching, your hands are so busy, that tactile need isn't there. And so I'm able to relax far more while using my hands in this way. I don't have that anxious attachment, this attachment from whatever device has taken over my life."

People respond to something in their hands. They appreciate the textures and colors of the yarn, the warmth and feeling of creating something. With each stitch or movement, it feels like everything is OK in the world at that moment.

While there is a fair amount of research on the benefits of touch, there is little evidence on the effect of specifically touching yarn or similar textiles on our overall health and well-being. One study published more than a century ago reported that people who were asked to touch (with their eyes closed) soft and smooth fabrics found those pleasant, while stiff, rough, and coarse textures were unpleasant.

Still, the feeling of comfort touching the yarns gives people and allowing them to focus and complete a project cannot be underestimated. Most yarn texture is soft and smooth to the touch, so while the research done is more than a century old, it's hard to imagine a similar study done today would yield wildly different results.

Finding a Creative Outlet

Both Blount and Downey love the activity and movement of embroidery and cross-stitching, and through the process, they discovered unexpected side benefits. For Downey, embroidery brought creativity back into her life, something she admitted was desperately lacking. Today, she has an exhibit made up of 270 pieces of work in a museum.

"It's slow. It's focused. It's repetitive, which I really like. And it's creative, especially when you're making your own work versus using patterns. You really have to spend some time being creative and coming up with things, and I love how it sort of cracked me open creatively."

Downey isn't alone in how she feels after doing embroidery work. In a study of more than thirty-five hundred knitters published in the *British Journal of Occupational Therapy*, 81 percent of respondents with depression reported feeling happy after knitting, while more than half reported feeling "very happy."

Soon, Downey found herself thinking differently about everything. She always identified as an artist, activist, and community builder, but as a queer feminist who is also anti-racist, anti-capitalist, and highly political, she wanted to use her platform as the founder of Badass Cross Stitch to create a more equitable world. According to Downey, her art generally tackles what she calls "the big three" systems of oppression: white supremacy, patriarchy, and capitalism.

It didn't take long for others to notice her and her work, and soon they began asking her to teach them how to stitch too. Downey realized this presented an opportunity to teach the benefits of embroidery while building much-needed community.

"The way I construct the events is an opportunity to

meet new people and, like, really meet new people, not like a networking event. This is something where, at the end of every workshop, people are exchanging phone numbers and making plans to hang out again. I think that's fucking magic for adults to go to a two-hour workshop and literally walk away with other people's phone numbers who they want to hang out with."

This part is just as important to Downey as the physical experience of stitching. She's successfully figured out how to do what she loves but also inject her passion for social justice issues with community.

Blount agrees the community-building aspect of embroidery can be especially beneficial. As she works with clients in her practice, especially during the intake process, she always asks them who is in their community to lean on for support. "If they can't name anyone, their first priority is to begin to identify those people who will have their back," she said. "Our community is critical."

That's not to say some people aren't apprehensive when they first try this type of embroidery or meet-ups.

If you've never touched a skein of yarn or tried to form a French knot, let alone more complicated knots, feeling nervous is understandable. You want to enjoy the feeling of your hand and wrists moving and the texture of the yarns on your skin and not be nervous about whether you're doing it right. You may want to use these community events to learn how to start or get better.

Downey is a master event planner, and she thinks through all these scenarios and concerns. She makes the experience fun and creates icebreakers so participants are laughing and relaxing and learning along the way. Once they start stitching and hands are moving, conversations flow effortlessly.

At the end of each event, Downey has everyone share three things as an intentional ending:

* One word that describes how you feel
* One thing you learned today
* One thing you're going to do tomorrow to change the world

The words people share are *connected, calm, focus, empower, empowered.* "The words that come out of it show the transformation from what happened when they walked in hours ago," Downey said. "And it gives them an opportunity to see that and feel that in their bodies and acknowledge it."

──────────── TRY IT ────────────

1 EXPERIMENT. If you're new to handiwork like embroidery or crocheting, experiment with different types to see what you enjoy the most. You may find handling one hook to crochet is easier than using a pair of needles to knit, while others prefer using a hoop to hold on to as they use needle and threads to cross-stitch.

2 FIND A COMMUNITY. While you can learn from online tutorials and books, it's a lot more fun to learn from others. As both Blount and Downey attest, finding your community

can be key to learning a new activity that is not only good for your mind and body but also good for your soul.

3 PROCESS OVER PERFECTION. Remember, it's not about the product but about the journey. Make mistakes, unravel threads and yarn, start again, try something new. Don't let yourself get hung up on what the final piece will look like. Instead, take advantage of the mental and physical health benefits this activity affords, and enjoy it for what it is.

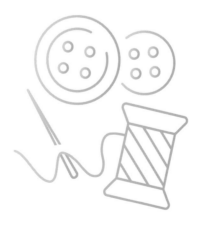

(7)

Let Your Worries Float Away

When Mark Smithivas, an entrepreneur based in Chicago, tried floatation therapy in his thirties, he was pursuing what he calls "mind-expanding" therapies. He thought floatation could help with creative breakthroughs.

"It is based on the concept of sensory deprivation, sort of like a natural psychedelic experience, so I was keen to try and see what would happen," Smithivas said. He compared floating to a massage "since it forces you to take a break from the normal daily routine and get in touch with your own thoughts and feelings."

Comparing floatation therapy, or floats, to massage isn't uncommon, but Dr. David Berv, a chiropractic sports physician, diplomate in acupuncture, and chief experience officer at the Float Zone in Richmond, Virginia, says the key difference is nobody is touching you during a float—just the water.

Berv had a thriving clinical practice when he was diagnosed with multiple sclerosis and suffered his first episode, which rendered him disabled for months. His brother recommended he try a "float" during a visit in Colorado. Berv had never even heard of floatation therapy but was willing to try it.

"I get into this fiberglass tank nine feet long by five feet wide with ten inches of skin-temperature salt water in it," Berv explained. "I get out of the tank after an hour and I'm like, oh my god, I can't believe how good I feel."

From the lens of a musculoskeletal specialist, Berv said he could see where this type of experience would be amazing for so many different applications. He decided to get a tank for his home, and after floating daily for a few years and noticing the many mind and body benefits, he decided to open a float center in Richmond and leave a twenty-year career in clinical practice.

How Floatation Works

Floatation therapy has origins with sensory deprivation, and while it does remove the senses, it also enhances them.

"Floatation-REST (Reduced Environmental Stimulation Therapy) reduces sensory input to the nervous system through the act of floating supine in a pool of water saturated with Epsom salt," according to a research study led by Dr. Justin Feinstein. "The float experience is calibrated so that sensory signals from visual, auditory, olfactory, gustatory, thermal, tactile, vestibular, gravitational and proprioceptive channels are minimized, as is most movement and speech."

Feinstein opened the first and only float lab in the country:

the Float Clinic and Research Center at the Laureate Institute for Brain Research in Tulsa, Oklahoma. While the research around the benefits of floatation is still in the infancy stage compared to studies of other types of therapies, *Time* magazine covered Feinstein and floatation in a feature and noted he and his team are seeing that floating tamps down anxiety in the brain in a way that rivals some prescription drugs and meditation.

While some clients are curious about the benefits of floatation therapy, most come to Berv's floatation clinic specifically to relieve stress and anxiety. First-time visitors watch an orientation video and then enter a private room with a shower to rinse off and a float tank with ten inches of ninety-four-degree Fahrenheit water. That's the approximate temperature of your skin at its most relaxed state, according to Berv.

The tank is filled with Epsom salt too. A lot of Epsom salt.

"You're using the largest organ of your body, namely your skin, to send a message to the brain to relax the entire body," Berv explained. "Secondly, and perhaps even most importantly, there are one thousand pounds of Epsom salt, or magnesium sulfate, dissolved in that ten inches of water."

Two things are happening as a result of the use of that magnesium sulfate, according to Berv.

"You're floating effortlessly, like a cork, because of the density of salt, which is denser than the Dead Sea. You are removing gravity from the equation."

Why is this important? Our brains spend so much time assessing our place in space. For example, when we enter the floatation tank, our brains are thinking, *Is this a danger to me?*

Am I going to fall over and hit my face? Am I going to drown? The brain is trying to make sense of the situation using all our senses: smell, taste, touch, sight, and sound. But when we remove gravity from the equation, we now allow the brain, which spends so much time with all that other stuff, to focus on other things.

The second thing that happens is the person in the tank is absorbing the magnesium through their skin. Magnesium sulfate is a chemical compound made up of magnesium, sulfur, and oxygen. According to some research, magnesium increases serotonin (the happiness or relaxation hormone) production in your brain.

Rhonda Mattox, MD, a board-certified physician in psychiatry and neurology, includes Epsom salt among the tools in her toolbox that can be useful for patients with a number of conditions, including anxiety, according to an article published in *Real Simple*.

You can float with the lid either closed or open. Some people, like Berv, enjoy floating in the dark, lid closed, and in silence. Others, like me, prefer keeping the lid open, calm music playing in the background, and lights on. Berv reminds clients it's *their* experience, so they can do whatever is most comfortable for them.

Once you're floating and have eliminated gravity, thanks to the Epsom salt and temperature of the water, you will feel like you're floating in a cloud. As a result, your brain is free from having to worry about anything, so this becomes a potent reset for the brain, Berv said.

According to Feinstein's research, study participants

reported significant reductions in stress, muscle tension, pain, depression, and negative affect, accompanied by a significant improvement in mood characterized by increases in serenity, relaxation, happiness, and overall well-being.

Many people report the effects are immediate, and Berv said many sleep like a baby that same night. The emotional benefits, he added, tend to last longer than the physical benefits.

"The more often you float, the longer those benefits last," Berv noted. "So if you float on a regular basis, that feeling might last a week, ten days, two weeks. For some people, even longer than that."

———————————— TRY IT ————————————

1. First, decide what you want to get out of the experience. Is it pain relief, anxiety relief, to feel calmer, or to clear your head to allow other thoughts to enter your headspace? Be clear with your intention.

2. After doing some research of floatation centers near you, check out the types of tanks each offers so you can decide whether you'd be comfortable in that environment. If you tend to get claustrophobic, for example, make sure the center has tanks where you can keep the lid open and lights on.

3. Also, note some appointments are available for sixty or ninety minutes. For first timers, it's advisable to book a shorter time period. Keep in mind, you can get out of the tank at *any* time.

④ Before your appointment, Berv recommends staying away from caffeine, excess fluids, or a large meal. Remember, you're going to be immobilized for about an hour, and the last thing you want is to need to take a bathroom break or to hear digestive noises throughout. Also, be on time so you're not rushing to your appointment. You want to arrive in as calm a state as possible so once you get into the tank, you can enjoy it.

⑤ If your first experience isn't what you were hoping, don't give up on floating. Instead, Berv recommends trying it during a different time or day of the week. If you went in the evening, try it in the morning or midday. If you went during the week, try it on the weekend. Each experience will be different, but finding when you can enjoy the experience the most will make a big difference.

8

Different Strokes

W hen our bodies ache, it's hard for our minds not to feel the ache too.

Muscles get locked with tension, and that tension reverberates through the entire body. The kneading and stroking movements of a massage, especially from an experienced massage therapist, can release these tensions, help us relax, and enhance our well-being. Part of the reason is what happens when hands touch our bodies—it goes beyond simply unknotting those tense muscles. Massage helps stimulate oxygen flow, which also helps increase our focus and concentration.

The power of intentional touch cannot be underestimated. While some might consider massage a luxury, the reality is it can be a powerful and long-lasting self-care activity.

KJ Hardy, a Chicago-based therapist, has long appreciated

and enjoyed the healing touch of a massage. She has been seeing the same massage therapist for more than fifteen years. "She knows my body and is very intuitive," Hardy told me. "I know I need a massage when I find myself feeling anxious and/or when I start to feel some kinks in my body."

Awareness of the mind-body connection is finding its way into the fields of medicine and integrative health care as more research shows the effects of massage are more than skin deep. Also, massage is becoming more widely available. Where you used to have to book a massage at a wellness resort or luxury spa, you can now book a therapist to come to your home or office, schedule an appointment at a local massage clinic, or even pop in without an appointment at an airport or while walking a trade show.

Hardy typically sees her massage therapist six times a year and is such a huge proponent of massages that she extols their virtue to anyone who will listen. After a massage, she said, your body and mind will thank you, and you'll find yourself booking the next one immediately.

Mark Smithivas, a busy Chicago-based entrepreneur, gets massages as a way to combat how he feels from sitting all day in front of a computer. Aside from the benefits of working out the kinks and feeling more blood flowing throughout his limbs and extremities, Smithivas said he enjoys the time on the massage table and the ability to detach from anything else going on in his life while he's getting a massage.

"It feels like 'me' time and a chance to enjoy the next sixty to ninety minutes in bliss," Smithivas said. He admitted that the post-massage effect can be fleeting if he knows he's in a rush to get to another appointment. Still, during that time on the table or on the floor if he's getting a Thai massage—his favorite kind—he can let go and sometimes even fall asleep.

There's a scientific reason we feel good during and after a massage. Massage therapy has been shown to lower stress, decrease anxiety, and reduce irritability. One study on massage found that levels of the stress hormone cortisol dropped 31 percent following a rubdown, while levels of feel-good hormones like dopamine and serotonin increased roughly 30 percent.

According to the Mayo Clinic, while more research is needed to confirm the benefits of massage, some studies have found massage to be helpful for a host of other issues, including the following:

* Anxiety
* Digestive disorders
* Fibromyalgia
* Headaches
* Insomnia related to stress
* Low back pain
* Myofascial pain syndrome
* Nerve pain
* Soft tissue strains or injuries
* Sports injuries
* Temporomandibular joint pain
* Upper back and neck pain

Unwinding Different Types of Massages

However, not all massages are the same. Massage is a general term for pressing, rubbing, and manipulating your skin, muscles, tendons, and ligaments, according to Mayo Clinic. It may range from light stroking to deep pressure and can be customized to your needs and time constraints.

For example, if you have pain in your neck, researchers from the University of Washington School of Public Health and the Group Health Research Institute in Seattle found that several sixty-minute massages per week for four weeks were more effective in treating chronic neck pain than fewer or shorter sessions. Another study found that short periods of relaxation, even just ten minutes of massage or relaxation, may be psychologically and physiologically regenerative and that the effect is even more pronounced with massage.

The most common types of massage are as follows:

* *Swedish massage,* which uses long strokes, kneading and deep circular movements, vibration, and tapping. It's considered a gentle form of massage.
* *Deep tissue massage,* which uses more forceful strokes to target the deeper layers of muscles and connective tissue.
* *Sports massage,* which is similar to a Swedish massage but geared toward people involved in sports to aid in preventing or treating injuries.

Customizing your experience isn't difficult and makes it more likely you'll be satisfied with the experience overall.

Runners, for example, might opt for a runner's massage since that type of massage will focus primarily on the lower body, such as the back, legs, and feet, and may incorporate muscle therapy lotion with cooling properties to help ease inflammation.

Thai massage is a little different from other types of massages in which you lie on a massage bed while a massage therapist uses oil and kneads your muscles and pressure points. During a Thai massage, you remain clothed (best to wear loose clothing), and the practitioner uses stretching and pulling techniques to help your body relieve tension and improve circulation. It's a more active-oriented type of massage, which is why it's also referred to as *assisted yoga* by some.

Hot stone massage uses smooth or flat heated stones to help you relax and ease those tense muscles. The stones, usually made of basalt, are heated to between 130 and 145 degrees and strategically placed along your spine or on your stomach and chest.

Prenatal massage is intended for expectant mothers and focuses on spots where pregnant women most frequently experience pain and discomfort as their pregnancy progresses.

Some therapists are adding different offerings to appeal to a larger group experiencing specific ailments that can benefit from the power of massage. Oncology massage uses gentle, gliding strokes meant to induce relaxation and pressure and can be adjusted based on the cancer client's needs.

While scheduling regular massages isn't financially plausible for everyone, scheduling one when you feel you can really benefit from a massage can go a long way to improving your mental health. But if time or finances don't allow it, a few tools at home can be beneficial too. A foam roller can alleviate pain in larger muscles, and electronic devices like a massage gun or massage chair can help by going a bit deeper since they vibrate faster. Even a tennis ball on the ground can help relieve some tension around your hips.

Or if you have a trusted partner at home willing to give you a massage, take them up on it! Sometimes all you need is a few good strokes to help calm your body and mind.

──────────────── TRY IT ────────────────

1. Ask someone you trust, whether it's a health-care provider or friends, for recommendations based on what type of massage you're seeking. Most states regulate massage therapists, so there's no need to be shy in asking potential therapists if they're licensed, certified, or registered and what type of training or experience they have. Once you find a therapist, ask what each session costs, and see if your insurance might cover it. Not all insurance plans cover massage, but some do, so it's worth asking.

2. One of the things Hardy loves about massages is you can control how you show up or participate. If you want to keep your clothes on, keep them on. If you don't want to talk, there's no need to talk. If you're finding the massage is too hard or too soft, let the therapist know so they can adjust. Typically, people undress (you can remove your undergarments or keep them on—it's totally up to you, and your therapist will

not judge you either way) and cover themselves with a sheet while the therapist is out of the room. However, you can still get a massage fully clothed and seated in a chair if that's your preference.

3 Depending on the length of time and type of massage, a therapist might engage other senses in addition to touch. They might apply essential oils (be sure to let your therapist know if you're allergic to any ingredients), play calming music, and dim the lights.

4 Finally, a massage could last ten minutes or ninety minutes, but no matter what kind of massage you get, the only thing you need to do is relax and let the therapist do their job.

5 If you have someone at home willing to give you a massage, start by trying to replicate a massage studio. Have some massage oil at hand (with your favorite fragrance), dim the lights, and choose a soft space like a bed or sofa. If you opt for the floor, add some pillows in spots where you'd like to alleviate pressure, such as your neck or lower back. Let the other person know what part of your body you want them to focus on and if the pressure they're using is too hard or too soft.

9

Scrub It Out

Most people don't love to clean or organize their home. Many of us typically view any cleaning activity as a chore rather than relaxing or meditative. However, some people actually *do* find some chores meditative and look forward to them. For those people, intentionally cleaning or organizing their spaces allows them to take control of something in their lives they can (positively) effect, forces their brain to take a break, and lets them clear their mind, which sometimes allows creativity to come into play (not always, but the break for the mind is a nice bonus).

Gail Adduci Gogliotti, LCPC, BC-DMT, a Chicago-based clinical counselor and dance/movement therapist with Kinesphere Counseling, understands the appeal of cleaning and organizing to some clients and looks at it from the perspective of how the brain organizes situations. It's not uncommon for some people to go on cleaning sprees when they're feeling really overwhelmed or stressed out or procrastinating because they don't want to deal with an issue they're facing.

"If your brain is cluttered with thoughts, it's very difficult to function externally," Adduci Gogliotti explained. "If you look at that inner/outer connection, what is happening internally is affected by what's happening externally and vice versa. If your external space feels calm or feels decluttered, it naturally will impact your body's ability or your mind's ability to feel more organized."

In other scenarios, clutter and disorganization themselves cause stress. Owner of the professional organizing firm Get Neat, Get Knox in Chicago, Jenifer Knox told me clutter and disorganization use our energy in a way we don't realize. "It's like having a project that you know has to be done (returning a phone call, paying bills, writing that term paper), yet there's no deadline so that project continues to take up mental energy," Knox explained. "Think about that pile of papers on the kitchen counter: 'I need to do something about that' is a constant internal refrain. Once that clutter is addressed and resolved, there is a sense of calm and accomplishment."

Knox helps clients create organized systems so they can get through their days using less energy and less stress. She likes to think of it as living more efficiently. "By creating systems, you (and everyone in your home) knows where the lightbulbs and batteries are kept. Sports uniforms. Music instruments. Cameras. Chargers. Permission slips," Knox noted. "When everything in your home has a place, you and the rest of the household members can find what is needed without thinking or having to ask anyone (usually Mom, right?). This helps to reduce that mental workload."

While having a clean and organized home is ideal, there is another benefit to the act of cleaning and organizing, according to Adduci Gogliotti: it helps us process things all jumbled in our heads or puts us into a different headspace.

As humans, we naturally like to intellectualize and rationalize situations, and that's where we get kind of tangled up in our thoughts. When we're doing activities externally, like cleaning or other types of movement using touch, then we're taking our state of being into something else. "Your focus goes naturally to something that is organizational," Adduci Gogliotti added.

Cleaning doesn't always mean organizing. There is science to support the idea that we can get into a meditative state during everyday activities like vacuuming, washing dishes, or folding laundry.

According to researchers at Florida State University, fifty-one college students were told to mindfully wash dishes before completing tasks related to mindfulness, affect, and experiential recall.

The study found "those who focused on the smell of the soap, the warmth of the water, the feel of the dishes— reported a decrease in nervousness by 27 percent and an increase in mental inspiration by 25 percent. The control group, on the other hand, didn't experience any benefits."

So if you're feeling anxious or need to mull over something, perhaps giving Roomba a day off and pulling out that vacuum instead is a smarter choice. Unlike other activities that require your focused attention (like driving), vacuuming, folding laundry, or washing dishes allows you to feel what you're doing but the activity is secondary. You're *doing* something, but your attention can work through other things in the background. The physical sensation often feels satisfying too. As you wash dishes, you can enjoy the feeling of the warm water on your skin. As you're folding laundry, you can appreciate the texture of the fibers you're folding neatly. The vibration of the vacuum has a calming effect on your body.

The topic is getting national attention. Ellen Byron wrote an article for the *Wall Street Journal* on the subject of cleaning as a form of meditation. In her piece, she interviewed psychologist Craig Sawchuk, who said, "Mindful cleaning offers multiple health benefits, including relaxing the body, calming the brain and fostering a sense of accomplishment when the job is done." He added that in the context of all uncertainty, mindful cleaning affords us a simple, good, and tangible way to help build up our resiliency and act as a buffer against stressors around us.

TRY IT

It's natural not to think about cleaning and organizing as a form of meditation, but it's worth giving a shot to see if it's helpful. Knox understands the struggle some people have with their spaces, and getting started is often the hardest part. She's found that it can be helpful for some people to hire a professional organizer, even if it's for one session, so they can get started. Or they might find it's better to hire someone for a project or to schedule intermittent sessions with a personal coach to stay accountable.

For those who want to try it on their own, Knox and Adduci Gogliotti offer some recommendations:

1. Start small. Even cleaning out or organizing a kitchen drawer will leave you with a sense of accomplishment. Think about what is bothering you the most, and start there. What do you feel you can accomplish in the time you have available? Completing something, whether it's vacuuming one room or putting away the dishes, will make you feel good, and you get to enjoy the added bonus of a cleaner space!

2. Set a time limit, and allow twenty to thirty minutes at the end for cleanup, depending on the project. If you only have an hour, that may not be the best time to do a closet overhaul. Save big projects for a weekend, because you might find yourself more stressed if you can't finish something and are facing a bigger mess than when you started.

3. To help the overall process, sort items into like categories, and purge any duplicates or things you really don't use. Knox advises her clients to be ruthless here.

4. It's tempting to procrastinate and buy "just the right" organizing containers, but Knox doesn't recommend investing in any organizing items until you've sorted and purged and measured the space. Instead, she tells clients to consider using containers they already have, such as food storage containers or shoeboxes.

5 Take the trash out, and load donations into the car immediately. There is something to be said about the act of physically removing things that no longer serve you in life. In this case, it's in the form of stuff. But removing things from your physical space and seeing the results can be incredibly satisfying.

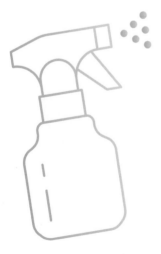

(10)

Wrapped in a Hug

Weighted blankets burst into the mainstream in 2017 thanks to social media and a successful Kickstarter campaign. Before then, their origin story dates back to the late 1990s, when an occupational therapist was using a weighted blanket with some of her mental health patients.

For those unfamiliar with this type of blanket, it looks like a regular blanket except that it's heavier because it's filled with high-density plastic or sand pellets (some blankets are filled with glass beads to provide gentle compression). They typically come in various weights, from five pounds to thirty pounds, and are available in the traditional bed sizes, from twin to king, or as a throw. In many cases, the blankets are machine washable and come in a variety of colors, making it easy to incorporate one into your bedding.

Some have described the weighted blanket on their body

as a warm hug, with the deep-pressure feeling comforting for many.

It could be argued that the hug machine was the impetus for the weighted blanket. Temple Grandin, PhD, an American scientist who also has autism, created a squeeze machine, also called a *hug box* or a *cow hug machine*, after observing cattle going through chutes at a family's farm. She noticed they would emerge from the chute relatively calmer. "The chute provided deep pressure stimulation against most of the animal's body."

She began experimenting by creating a squeeze machine (a deep-pressure device designed to administer pressure evenly through the body between two sideboards hinged in a V shape) to apply deep-touch pressure as a way to help reduce anxiety and nervousness and recruited college students to test the machine for five to ten minutes as a pilot study. She was attending college herself when she created the therapeutic, stress-relieving device. While the sample size was low, the results did show that deep-pressure stimulation seemed to decrease anxiety levels of those who used it compared to those who didn't use it.

In 1992, she published some of her findings based on her squeeze machine. In Grandin's report, "the 'squeeze machine' applies lateral, inwardly directed pressure to both lateral aspects of a person's entire body, by compressing the user between two foam-padded panels. Clinical observations and several studies suggest that deep touch pressure is therapeutically beneficial for both children with an autistic disorder and probably children with attention-deficit hyperactivity disorder."

"Pressure is calming to the nervous system," Grandin said during an interview with Colorado State University in 2015. She referenced products like the anxiety wrap or the Thundershirt for dogs as things that have helped both humans and animals. Other examples we might be familiar with to illustrate this feeling include compression clothing like weighted vests or even compression socks.

The weighted blanket isn't a machine, but the weight helps apply that same type of deep-pressure stimulation found in the hug machine.

"The pressure a weighted blanket provides when someone is trying to relax into sleep can be comforting," Dr. Lynette Schneeberg, a behavioral sleep psychologist and Fellow of the American Academy of Sleep Medicine, said in a *USA Today* article on the rise in popularity of weighted blankets in early 2019. "People like the feeling of getting a hug or a massage. Sleeping under a weighted blanket provides a similar feeling."

Sensing an opportunity and on the heels of a hotly contested presidential election where anxiety levels among many Americans were riding high, a company called Gravity pursued a Kickstarter campaign to sell its Gravity Blanket on April 26, 2017.

According to its Kickstarter campaign product description, "Gravity is a premium-grade, therapeutic weighted blanket that harnesses the power of deep touch stimulation to gently distribute deep pressure across your body. Engineered to be around 10% of your body weight, Gravity helps relax the nervous system by simulating the feeling of being held or hugged. This increases serotonin and melatonin levels and decreases cortisol levels—improving your mood and promoting restful sleep at the same time. All without ever filling a prescription."

Perhaps it was the promising language that a simple blanket could do so much to help us sleep or ease our anxiety or the timing of it, but the campaign raised $100,000 within the first hour.

Time magazine called the Gravity Blanket one of the fifty best inventions of 2018 because it eases anxiety.

Weighted blankets are something many occupational therapists have been using for years as a form of sensory integration therapy, especially with children who have trouble processing their senses. They stimulate those patients' senses of touch, helping their brains adapt, which is thought to help them better control their emotions and boost their mental health.

While there is no shortage of anecdotal support for weighted blankets, much of the research to date has been focused on their use with psychiatric patients or children on the autism spectrum or with ADHD. One study found the use of weighted blankets to be a safe and potentially effective way to help individuals in a psychiatric facility manage anxiety.

"This study found that use of a 14-pound or 20-pound weighted blanket or a 5-pound lap pad for approximately 20 minutes significantly decreased anxiety and pulse rate in adults experiencing anxiety in an inpatient mental health unit. The comparison group, who did not use a weighted blanket or lap pad, did not exhibit a statistically significant reduction in pulse rates or anxiety scores," the study concluded.

When we're feeling anxious, our autonomic nervous systems—which control basic bodily functions such as breathing, digestion, sweating, and shivering—prepare our bodies for stress or rest, according to Penn Medicine, and this is referred to as our fight-or-flight response.

"The pressure of weighted blankets puts your autonomic nervous system into 'rest' mode, reducing some of the symptoms of anxiety, such as a quickened heart rate or breathing," Penn Medicine continues. "This can provide an overall sense of calm."

Annette Becklund, therapist and the lead author of another published study, has worked extensively in mental health hospitals and has seen firsthand the positive impact of weighted blankets on patients. "I watched people who were going to be put into restraints not have to be put into restraints because we offered them the blankets first," Becklund said in a *Popular Science* article.

While research in nonpsychiatric spaces isn't as readily available to support the use of weighted blankets as a way to calm the body and mind, what research is being done and published seems to be positive. One study showed that 63 percent of participants reported lower anxiety after use of a thirty-pound weighted blanket in a lying down position, while 78 percent preferred the weighted blanket as a calming modality.

Seeing firsthand the benefits weighted blankets can have

on individuals, therapists like Becklund don't hesitate to recommend them, with the caveat that each person should consult with a physician about medical concerns first and not buy one that's too heavy.

————————————— TRY IT —————————————

1. Ask your health-care provider if using a weighted blanked might be helpful and if there are any medical concerns. For some people, a weighted blanket might feel claustrophobic, and it might cause problems for people with certain medical conditions. Also, it's important to speak to a child's physician before using weighted blankets as some manufacturers discourage their use for children under the age of ten. Note that when using one, you must have the dexterity to lift the blanket off your body when necessary.

2. Experts recommend using a blanket that is 10 percent of your body weight, give or take a pound or two.

3. Blankets range from about five to twenty-five pounds and come in many different colors, styles, and textures. Choose the weight and texture that feels the most soothing to encourage you to use it as often as you want or need to.

4. Some experts recommend using a weighted blanket for about twenty to thirty minutes. Some people enjoy using them as part of their sleep routine or when they want to relax after a long and stressful day. It's really up to you and what makes you feel calm and relaxed.

5. Thanks to their recent popularity, it's easy to find weighted blankets at most major retailers and at different price points. Depending on the size and retailer, expect to pay between $50 and $300, with most around the low to mid-$100 range.

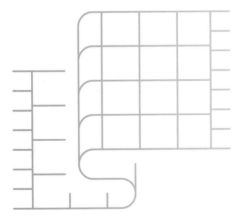

Letters of Gratitude

Sending a thank-you card to a friend or expressing gratitude is more than just good manners. It feels good, for the sender and receiver.

"We are always exploring methods which can improve health, but no one ever looked at a series of letters to see if it benefits the author's well-being," noted Dr. Steven Toepfer, an associate professor of human development and family studies at Kent State University. "We know people who receive letters of gratitude benefit, but what about the authors? Will you feel better by writing letters of gratitude? Are multiple letters better than a single composition?"

One of Toepfer's studies examined the effects of writing letters of gratitude on three primary qualities of well-being: happiness (positive affect), life satisfaction (cognitive evaluation), and depression (negative affect). Gratitude was also assessed. Results from the research indicated that writing letters of gratitude increased participants' happiness and life satisfaction while decreasing depressive symptoms.

The study participants were divided into two groups. One group wrote a letter of gratitude to anyone they wanted each week for three weeks, and the other group did not. The letter had to include something important to the writer, not simply a generic "thank you for the gift" kind of message.

"As they wrote, up to three letters, results showed increasing benefits," Toepfer noted. "The more letter writing people did, the more they improved significantly on happiness and life satisfaction. The new and potentially important finding is that depressive symptoms decreased. By writing these letters—15 to 20 minutes each, once a week for three weeks to different people—well-being increased significantly."

Just as significant, the group that did not write letters but filled out the questionnaires about their well-being early in the study process found their well-being did not change.

"What we come away with from this study is that if you are looking to increase your well-being through intentional activities, take 15 minutes three times over three weeks and write letters of gratitude to someone," Toepfer said in an article written by Emily Vincent for Kent State University.. "You'll feel better on those three variables. There is a cumulative effect, too. If you write over time, you'll feel happier, you'll feel more satisfied, and if you're suffering from depressive symptoms, your symptoms will decrease."

Not Another Quick Digital Note

Sending an email or quick text thanking someone for something is lovely and likely appreciated by the recipient, but nothing beats taking the time to write something by hand. Also, when we're emailing or texting someone, it's not usually to thank the person but because we need or want something.

A physical card, even if it simply says thank you on the cover, is pretty. It can be elegant, colorful, or formal, but it's physical, unlike a quick text that will be seen in one second and deleted the next.

Even if you feel your handwriting is atrocious, the gratitude sentiment will go a lot further and for a few reasons.

1. The physical act of sitting down and taking the time to compose and write your letter matters. You're thinking about your recipient and about what this person did that brought you joy. It doesn't have to be a big, momentous thing either. It could be that the person took time out of their day to lend a helping hand or you wanted to acknowledge or recognize something they did for someone else. When you put it in writing, the physical act of writing it rather than shooting off a text gives more weight to the message.

2. In our digital age, getting anything other than bills or direct mail solicitations via snail mail is almost unheard of, so receiving a handwritten card will definitely stand out. And your recipient won't note your

atrocious handwriting but the fact that you took the time to write and send it.

3. You can inject your personality into the card. You can choose a card that is simple, formal, funny, or sentimental. It can be sent in a colorful envelope or not. The card or stationery itself can be part of the whole experience.

If writing thank-you letters is so easy and inexpensive and can lift our moods, why is it such a challenge for some of us? Many of us find we're too concerned with getting the words and intention right or how our recipients will feel when they receive our note. So instead of taking the time to sit down and craft a kind note, even if it'll only take a minute or two, we don't because we don't always know what to say or how the person who is to receive it will feel, according to another research study.

"Expressing gratitude improves well-being for both expressers and recipients, but an egocentric bias may lead expressers to systematically undervalue its positive impact on recipients in a way that could keep people from expressing gratitude more often in everyday life," according to the research findings.

But the study showed how misguided these feelings are.

As part of the study, participants wrote gratitude letters and then predicted how surprised, happy, or awkward recipients would feel. On the flip side, the recipients then reported how receiving an expression of gratitude actually made them feel. Those who sent the letters significantly underestimated how surprised recipients would be about why expressers were grateful, overestimated how awkward recipients would feel, and underestimated how positive recipients would feel.

The intention and mindfulness involved with letter writing are what make it so powerful.

─────────────── TRY IT ───────────────

Writing a gratitude letter can be a whole-body experience. It's hard to do it in haste. Unlike typing on a computer or recording a message by phone, where you sometimes don't even have to glance at a screen to know what you're going to type or say, you have to pull out a pen and paper to write a note.

1. Unless you have a stash of notecards and stamps at the ready, take a trip to a stationery shop and let your eyes feast on the beautiful accoutrements. Touch the beautiful stationery, and appreciate the smoothness of the writing instruments.

2. Once you've decided which stationery to use, take a moment to jot down some initial thoughts about why you're grateful. This process can bring about joy as you think about the person who will be the receiver of your gratitude. Take yourself out of the habit of whipping out quick messages and sound bites and checklists. Your note doesn't need to be a laundry list or love note. It can simply reference one thing for which you're grateful.

3. Once you have a clear idea of what you want to say, write a

few sentences (or more, if you wish). During this process, you can incorporate other senses like taste and smell if you want to savor the moment with a hot cup of tea or coffee or snack on some biscuits. Play some relaxing music in the background. Enjoy the whole experience, and don't rush.

4. Want a more social experience? Consider joining a correspondence club or writing society where members of the community gather on a regular basis to write letters, postcards, and note cards together. Some stationery shops or book shops organize these groups as well, and if there isn't one near you, why not start one? To get ideas on how some are organized (or to see if one is available near you), check out the Letter Writing Societies + Clubs page of letterseals.com. For example, the Correspondence Club of Bloomington, Indiana, began when Addison Rogers wanted to introduce more people to the power of sending and receiving mail. He brings the stationery and writing instruments for free, and if people need a stamp, he sells those at cost. He even offers to deliver the letters to the post office when the event is over. Rogers and his friends meet every Tuesday at locations such as bars, coffee shops, or restaurants.

A Purrfect Way to De-Stress

That purr you hear when a kitten comes near you at a pet shelter sometimes feels like exactly what you both need. And those cuddles are the best. When cats and kittens rub up against you and nudge their sweet faces into your hands, it's their body language saying, "please pet me."

Every week, Jim Horst looks forward to his volunteer time at Harmony House for Cats, a cats-only no-kill shelter near his home that he calls his happy place. Unfortunately, his wife and son are allergic to cats, but he and his daughter aren't. And since they both love cats, she encouraged him to start volunteering at their local shelter. He began going twice a week to play with the cats, manage volunteers, give orientations, and do transport runs to the vet. During the pandemic, when volunteers weren't permitted in the shelter, he kept volunteering as a transport.

"Cats are very much like people and have very individual personalities," Horst told me. Over the years, he's learned to read their cues and become friends with approximately seventy-five cats. "Like people, some cats like you, others would prefer you leave them alone."

He calls his weekly visits the best part of his week. "A good cat friend will purr for you, give you head boops, and cuddle sometimes," he added. He feels many cats enjoy the attention of petting and cuddles since it mimics some grooming behaviors.

For Horst, volunteering at the cat shelter means more than just spending time with the cats. He considers them friends and enjoys the time he gets with them. Sure, some can be moody at times, but generally, he says, they're glad to see each other.

Volunteering, in general, can be a great salve for our minds and bodies. Many people report how much they enjoy the camaraderie they feel when they spend time helping others, including animals like cats and dogs. It wards off loneliness and depression and gives them purpose. Someone is depending on them and their care.

That simple human touch can go a long way in helping counteract the negative effects of anxiety, stress, and anger. Horst looks forward to his weekly visits with his feline friends. One of the reasons he feels spending time with cats or dogs at a shelter can have the power to be calming in our lives is that the engagement is a purely physical and emotional connection with no back talk or difficult conversations.

"A human's relationship with an animal is relatively

uncomplicated," he added. "If you know how to interpret their body language, you can tell what they are feeling and many times tell exactly what they want."

Research has shown that simply petting a dog lowers a person's level of the stress hormone cortisol. One study showed students who petted a cat or dog for ten minutes experienced momentary stress relief.

Additional insights shared by Johns Hopkins Medicine note that just having a pet, like a dog, lowers one's cortisol levels, and the social interaction between people and their dogs actually increases levels of the feel-good hormone oxytocin (the same hormone that bonds mothers to babies).

Another benefit? Having a pet or being around animals and petting them helps lower your blood pressure.

"The cortisol-lowering and oxytocin-boosting benefits of petting also help keep your blood pressure at bay," the article noted. "Petting and holding an animal allows you to appreciate the beauty of nature," Jeremy Barron, MD, medical director of the Beacham Center for Geriatric Medicine at Johns Hopkins, shared in the piece. "It's relaxing and transcendental."

NIH News in Health, a monthly newsletter from the National Institutes of Health, reports that pets can help decrease stress, improve heart health, and help children with their emotional and social skills. In addition to the research citing human-animal interactions showing a decrease of cortisol and lowering of blood pressure, the February 2018 newsletter stated that other studies have found animals can reduce loneliness, increase feelings of social support, and boost your mood.

"There's not one answer about how a pet can help somebody with a specific condition," Dr. Layla Esposito, who oversees NIH's Human-Animal Inter-action Research Program, explained in the article. "Is your goal to increase physical activity? Then you might benefit from owning a dog. You have to walk a dog several times a day and you're going to increase physical activity. If your goal is reducing stress, sometimes watching fish swim can result in a feeling of calmness. So there's no one type that fits all."

TRY IT

1. Before you commit to a shelter to volunteer your time, visit several shelters you're interested in and ask questions. Ask how the pets waiting for adoption live, what happens to the ones who don't get adopted, and whether there are opportunities that would fit your schedule and lifestyle.

2. Ask if you can volunteer a couple of times before committing to something longer term. When you have a chance to spend time at a shelter, consider how you interact with the animals. Simple acts like sitting down and letting them come to you first can be hard but will go a long way to establishing rapport with them. Try not to pet animals on top of their heads, which they might perceive as an aggressive act. If they seem comfortable, try scratching underneath their chin, and feel how they react to your calming movements toward them.

3 If you don't have the ability or schedule flexibility to volunteer, perhaps you can offer to foster pets until they find their forever homes.

4 If you're looking to adopt a pet, first offer to pet sit the kind of animal you're hoping to adopt. Unlike a volunteer gig, adopting a pet is a long-term commitment. Again, you'll want to make sure you understand what it takes to bring a pet into your life.

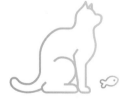

(13)

Mind Games

A jigsaw puzzle on a dining room table tempts you to see if you can place one more piece in its rightful spot. A crossword puzzle makes you pause and think about what words could work. When Wordle took the world by storm in 2022, some neurologists weren't surprised. The online word game that gives players six chances to guess a randomly selected five-letter word is fun and challenging, and it's among the types of puzzles that cognitive scientists know can be great for brain health.

"Puzzles and games, especially those involving novelty, can stimulate and challenge key parts of the brain, including reasoning, language, logic, visual perception, attention and problem-solving," Douglas Scharre, MD, neurologist and professor at the Ohio State Wexler Medical Center, wrote for *Health & Discovery* on the university's website. The "use it or lose it" mentality that applies to muscles also applies to the brain. "Using your brain in any way is thought to build up new connections between nerve cells in the brain," Scharre added. "This increases your brain reserve, so to speak."

While some people might find puzzles and word games an effective way to de-stress, others may find them too stressful, causing more anxiety. For those who find playing a game of skill fun, successfully solving them can give them a sense of completion and achievement, and Scharre said that's valuable. "In their small way, these games can help individuals in the pursuit of happiness," he added.

Working on puzzles is a healthy distraction because it also requires our undivided attention, can help reduce stress, and enhances our memory. However, these benefits are not limited to word puzzles.

Melissa Blount, PhD, a licensed clinical psychologist, was waiting for her mom to come out of surgery due to complications from cancer and found herself stressing as she had her infant daughter with her. She kept thinking about all the hospital germs surrounding both of them while also worrying about what was happening with her mom. She visited the hospital gift shop and bought herself a jigsaw puzzle, mostly to take her mind off what was going on around her.

"I started doing puzzles in the lobby while I was waiting for the surgeon to come back," Blount told me. "And it was something that literally saved my life in that moment."

It turned out she could do a puzzle with one hand since she could still nurse her young daughter when needed or rock her when she was being fussy or needed to sleep. It wasn't something she had to learn, like crocheting. She was able to look for pieces in between breaks and put them in place. It was a way for her to manage the overwhelming situation at hand and keep her mind busy while allowing her to care for a little human at the same time.

While much of the research around puzzles centers around cognitive benefits such as preventing cognitive decline in aging, there is some evidence to suggest that leisure activities such as engaging in jigsaw puzzling could help people cope with stressors such as regulating distressing emotions.

"Jigsaw puzzling may provide two active ingredients (i.e., effective features) that benefit cognition: first, process-specific cognitive demands of jigsaw puzzling could contribute to an increased brain reserve and second, regulation of distressing emotions through jigsaw puzzling could prevent chronic stress states that can exert a negative impact on cognitive aging and dementia in the long term," one scientific study noted.

And then there are board games. While Shannan Hofman Bunting admits playing board games doesn't calm her, it is a great equalizer in many instances as it's one of the few things her family members, who range in age from fifteen to fifty-one, can do together and that they *all* like. "The friendly (mostly) competition and the collective focus provide a lot of great memories and a real opportunity for connection," Bunting told me. "Strategic board games cause you to use parts of your brain that don't always get accessed...but we really enjoy it as something we do together; even my college kid *wants* to sit around and play a game with us!"

Still, she thinks one of the best reasons activities like solving a puzzle or participating in a board game help calm the body and mind is they require concentration or attention on what you're doing, which means we have to filter out other distractions like phones. You're also touching the pieces, whether a jigsaw puzzle piece or board game piece, and considering your next move. "And depending on the game, you have an opportunity to transport yourself (even just a little) to another world created by the game," she added.

─────────────────── TRY IT ───────────────────

1 Some major daily newspapers still offer a daily crossword puzzle in their print issues, including the *New York Times*. There are also softcover crossword puzzle books if you want something that has several puzzles to try and want to keep around at home or in your bag. While you don't get the same tactile benefits of completing a game on paper, if you want something daily and online, try solving a crossword puzzle or word game like the *New York Times* online daily crossword puzzle or Wordle's word game.

2 Sudoku is a popular logic-based, combinatorial number-placement puzzle. To successfully complete the puzzle, you have to fill a nine-by-nine grid with digits so that each column, row, and three-by-three section contain the numbers between one and nine. Although digital versions are available, to enjoy the benefit of touch, seek out a printed version so you can use a pencil or pen for a tactile experience.

③ Jigsaw puzzles can be as easy or complicated as you'd like. Want something relatively easy that you can finish quickly? Choose puzzles with fewer tiles or pieces to place in order to complete the design. If you want something that will require more time and challenge, opt for puzzles with more pieces or more complicated designs that will be more difficult to assemble. Allow yourself the benefit of holding your jigsaw puzzle pieces and feeling the shape—it might help you find its home on the puzzle. Some people go a step further and frame their puzzle as artwork once they've completed it as a nice memory of their experience.

④ If you'd like to try playing cards or board games with friends or family, see if you can find a game that will appeal to your age group. Bunting and her family really like Ticket to Ride. According to the manufacturer, Ticket to Ride is a cross-country train adventure in which players collect and play matching train cards to claim railway routes connecting cities throughout North America. The longer the routes, the more points they earn, and additional points come to those who can fulfill their Destination Tickets by connecting two distant cities and to the player who builds the longest continuous railway. When going on road trips, Bunting brings a deck of cards to play euchre or the Monopoly card game.

(14)

Unbound

Sometimes it's smooth, and sometimes it's coarse. Sometimes it feels cool to the touch, and other times it feels warm and comforting.

Paper and handmade books can feel so calming.

I couldn't tell you the first time I fell in love with the feeling of paper, but Lesa Dowd, a Chicago-based bookbinder and conservator, reminds us that we've been around books since childhood. As babies and toddlers, many of us were read to, and once we were able, we'd help our readers by holding the book and turning its pages.

My love for different types of papers and their textures grew over the years as I was drawn to the vast range of journals available to write in. I loved how my pen would glide as I wrote on some pages and how a notebook with handmade paper felt as I carried it around. I would seek out Japanese stationery shops whenever I traveled so I could buy a new journal (or two or three).

Then I stumbled on a stationery shop near where I lived, and while I was admiring all the handmade papers in the retail section, I noticed the owner was teaching a class on bookbinding in the studio right behind the cash register counter.

Could I make my own book, using papers I chose, and use it for journaling? I signed up for a course and have made several journals since.

Bookbinding, I've since learned, can be a wonderfully delightful and calming experience and one that helps you create something you can use immediately. While it is possible to create a book where you can add pages, most people who do not do this as a career create a small book or journal for a specific purpose like a sketchbook or journal. Or they can create a book to hold family recipes or even a wedding program or guestbook. How one uses a book they create is as varied as the person creating it.

Dowd is a professional bookbinder and conservator, a person who repairs and preserves works of art. Dowd has worked in major libraries, has helped create exhibits and installations, and restores books for private clients. She's also taught classes on bookbinding techniques and creating different objects using paper.

Dowd started bookbinding as a means to explore her artistic inner self outside her daily job. "In this world of increasing digital media, I find the immersive and tactile nature of bookbinding most calming," she told me.

For those who've never tried something like bookbinding

or a paper-based activity, Dowd said it might appeal to people interested in channeling a different part of their brain since it's not just about making something with your hands but the need to be fully part of the experience.

Like what attracted Dowd to the artistic form, many of her students comment that they love using their hands to create something and appreciate the object for what it is not—it's not digital.

"I liken the art and craft of bookbinding to the world of slow fashion," Dowd explained. Or slow food. It's about getting back to the basics.

And like cooking, one thing has to be done before the next step. You can't put the cover on the book, for example, before folding the pages. You cannot stitch the pages, if it is a book you will be stitching together, if you don't fold the pages first. There are certain steps you need to do in order.

One also needn't be an artist to do this activity, although it might encourage more artistic exploration as one gains experience by creating more paper-based projects, whether they're journals or paper-wrapped boxes.

"Bookbinding is an excellent craft for the mental or nervous convalescent because it is a 'developing task,' by which I mean that the work begins with simple operations which gradually become more difficult and call for greater mental effort," wrote William Rush Dunton in his book published in 1918, *Occupation Therapy: A Manual for Nurses*. His book was written for nurses who provide occupational therapy or care to patients, and he dedicated an entire chapter to the power of bookbinding and paper.

Since paper is a material that is readily available and inexpensive, it's another great reason to use your hands to try a new activity like bookbinding.

Bookbinding as a process requires us to slow down. You have to think about the step you're doing before you can move to the next step. You have to slow life down in order to feel the paper in your hands, thread a needle through the crease of a fold to create a stitch, or glue the spine to hold sections of papers together before adding the cover.

Each touchpoint is important. Dowd also reminds us that not every book has to be complicated, nor does everything involving paper need to be a book.

"Book and paper arts are a really good way for people to tune out the outside world and become focused on something that's a very tactile thing," she said.

If you love the feeling of different types of paper and journals as I do, perhaps making a blank notebook you can journal in is a good fit for you. Or use a specific bookbinding stitch that allows your spine to lie flat so you can sketch or create an album to store your kids' school artwork or keepsake pictures. You can also cover existing books or make boxes using paper. You can fold paper and make origami or create envelopes to send mail. There is letterpress printing where you can print texts.

Bookbinding is just one thing you can do with paper. In all the years and classes Dowd has taught, she said there has never been a time someone left her class regretting having spent the time touching and engaging with paper.

"Bookbinding and the book and paper arts offer many

different levels of opportunity for people to slow down and enjoy a creative process that involves the senses."

———————————— TRY IT ————————————

1. If bookbinding or working with papers is new to you and you want to learn the technique, head to your local library. There is no shortage of books on…well…books! You'll find books on how to make books and different things you can make or create with paper.

2. If the local library offers slim pickings or you want to get a better idea of techniques, look for local in-person classes where you can work with an artist or professional. They can guide you as part of a smaller class or one-on-one and provide immediate feedback to help you with a specific project. Or you can also check out online classes. There are many YouTube videos with step-by-step tutorials.

3. Once you're ready to start a project, it's time to go shopping for or find your paper. When you're seeking out paper to work with, take your time. You're not simply choosing paper; allow yourself to experience it. Feel the texture in your hands. Is it smooth so when you use your writing instrument it'll feel like it's gliding across the page or rougher like handmade paper so your pen will feel some grooves as you write on it?

4. When Dowd works on a client project, she first considers why she's binding the book and how will it be used. If the book's content is blank, then she'll ask if its purpose is so the

user will draw, sketch, or write in it. If so, she'll select internal papers appropriate for the purpose with attention to how the paper feels in the hand, the sound it makes when pages are turned, and how it will respond to the intended media. "For covering a book, I select materials and papers that harmonize with the intended use," she added.

5. I love creating books that I use. At first, I didn't want to write in my journal because it took me hours to create it, and I just loved touching the cover, flipping the interior pages, and even smelling it. I didn't start writing until I realized I could do it *daily* if I used my book as my journal, as I had originally intended. And once I wrote in all the pages, I simply made myself a new journal. And that's the best part: now that I know how to do simple bookbinding, I can enjoy the tactile process over and over again, and I intentionally seek out papers I can use for my next project.

6. Finally, if you just don't have it in you to make a book but want to watch someone else make it, check out bitter melon bindery on YouTube (https ://www.youtube.com/c/bitter melonbindery/). Its YouTube channel is managed by Chanel, who invites viewers to her bookbinding studio. Her videos are meant to teach, inspire, and relax. With titles like "Cozy Bookbinding with Calming Piano" or "Bookbinding Brings Me Calm and Presence," it's a lovely way to watch someone create something by hand without chatter.

$$15$$

Connect the Mind and Body

Yoga is about breathing. It's meditation. It's poses and stretches. It's feeling your feet touch the ground. It calms your body. It calms your mind. It's all this and so much more.

When most people think about practicing yoga, they usually think about the downward-facing dog pose or sitting on a yoga mat with a yogi leading them through various poses. Sure, this is yoga too. Kind of.

"Yoga goes beyond just the movement. It is about meditation. It is about reflection, self-study," explained DuShaun Branch, founder of Sage Gawd Collective, a yoga and wellness business specialized in making yoga as accessible for people as possible. "Like thinking about the senses. This is something that I think about, and I do a lot of work with young people. Enticing your senses, being aware of your smells, your sounds, those kinds of things. That's all yoga as well."

Amy Guth often says yoga saved her life, and that's no hyperbole. Guth is a journalist and screenwriter/producer who has practiced yoga for sixteen years and is certified to teach yoga and meditation. But she wasn't always a fan of yoga. As an endurance runner, she admits yoga meant nothing to her prior to an accident that changed her life.

Guth was in a major car accident in the early 2000s, and after the big stuff healed, she was left with a high level of chronic pain and limited mobility. "When you're dealing with chronic pain, that's often all you can focus on, so I got into a pretty dark place," Guth told me.

It was a neighbor who was involved in yoga who finally encouraged her to attend a restorative/gentle hatha combination class.

"I only had an image of people twisting themselves into advanced poses, and so I resisted attending," she added. Finally, out of desperation, she went. "I was frustrated and near tears to see people around me seeming to so effortlessly move and bend and hold poses when I could barely sit up without pain. The instructor apparently sensed this and came over to my mat, instructing me to lie down, and she slid rolled towels and bolsters under my knees and elbows and whispered, 'Just be where you are today.' I fell asleep and woke up a long time later. The class was long over, and the instructor sat reading quietly. I apologized for dozing off, and she dismissed it with 'You seemed like you needed some rest.'"

That yoga teacher convinced Guth that yoga isn't a

pass-fail situation. Rather, yoga is in the doing, not in the achievement. Allowing yourself to feel your hands connect, to touch the ground when doing a pose or simply being. "She encouraged me to come back often, with no expectation other than lying there," she added. "I think that was the first time in my entire life anybody ever showed me radical acceptance like that, that it was okay to show up exactly how I was, that nobody wanted anything from me, and that my yoga practice was a matter of coming to my mat, not in how I could contort myself."

It's not unusual for people to not really know what the word *yoga* means, says Lisa Faremouth Weber, a yoga teacher who has taught over two thousand hours. Faremouth Weber is also completing a master of yoga studies program at Loyola Marymount University, focusing on yoga therapy, and is the founder of Heaven Meets Earth Yoga in Evanston, Illinois.

"*Yoga* means to yoke. The word *yoga* is 'yuj' in Sanskrit. The main practice of yoga is meditation," Faremouth Weber explained.

So is yoga downward-facing dog poses? Yes and no.

The purpose of yoga is to balance or connect the mind, body, and breath, according to Faremouth Weber. Too often, we choose to separate these things or consider them unconnected, but what many of us don't immediately recognize is that when one is affected or changes, it reflects in the others. If our minds are busy or things feel intense, our breathing changes and our bodies feel that as well. When our bodies are stiff because we're stressed, our minds and breathing are affected. You can quiet your breathing by quieting your mind, which you can do by quieting your body's activity. It's all connected, and proper yoga poses or asanas (the Sanskrit word for poses or postures of yoga) allow you to do this and are one aspect of the practice of yoga.

"If you want to sit down and close your eyes and breathe, you're doing yoga. If you want to go into child's pose, you're doing yoga," Faremouth Weber pointed out. "Yoga refers to your ability to be steadfast in whatever you're doing. Whether you're walking outside, whether you're doing the downward-facing dog, whether you're sitting and closing your eyes and breathing, you're specific in your focus. You're not just doing nothing. It has to do with the integration of your awareness, everything that is you: your body, your breath."

When Branch decided to start teaching yoga, her main motivation was to make space for people to rest and to make it more accessible, especially for people of color. "When I worked in higher ed full-time and saw my students being super stressed, I wanted to make space for them to breathe, to be and to rest."

Branch wants her students to realize yoga is a daily practice, and to really see the benefits, you need to practice when you *don't* need it for the times that you do. She understands we're busy and constantly on the go, which is why she recommends creating a tool kit of things you can immediately apply to your life when needed.

So when you're anxious or stressed out and barely breathing, Branch suggests actively breathing in through your nose and giving a big sigh out through your mouth. "That's a tool you can put into your tool kit. Also, in my classes, I always talk about just noticing your feet on the floor. That brings you presence. That's a tool that you can put into your tool kit."

There is no shortage of scientific research showing the positive effects of a regular yoga practice. One study reported the regular practice of yoga promotes strength, endurance, and flexibility and facilitates characteristics of friendliness, compassion, and greater self-control while cultivating a sense of calmness and well-being.

Results from another study show that "yogic practices enhance muscular strength and body flexibility, promote and improve respiratory and cardiovascular function, promote recovery from and treatment of addiction, reduce stress, anxiety, depression, and chronic pain, improve sleep patterns, and enhance overall well-being and quality of life."

Whatever your motivation to introduce yoga or resume the practice in your life, realize you can define it however you feel it best serves you. Allow yourself the beauty of grounding your body and mind in a way that reduces the noise in your head.

——————————— TRY IT ———————————

1. If you're just starting out, read a book about yoga, or try a gentle or basic yoga class at a local community center or gym where you can get expert instruction on the practice of yoga.

2. Branch recommends going online and searching platforms like Instagram to find people like you who are practicing yoga. If you're a Black woman or a plus-size woman, search for phrases like #blackgirlyoga or #plussizeyoga. Once you

start noticing more people like you who are practicing, "then go for a class with somebody who talks about teaching in an accessible way," she added.

3 If the idea of going to a class is too intimidating because you don't know the postures, watch YouTube videos until you get comfortable with the terms and postures, or join a class virtually as many are offered via Zoom.

4 Once you're ready, Faremouth Weber recommends reaching out to someone you feel has a solid understanding of what it means to practice yoga—beyond just doing the poses. You want to work alongside someone you can trust and who can guide you along the way.

5 And what if you fall during a pose? That's OK! Branch said, "It's OK to fall over! Again, we are not seeking perfection. This journey is yours to connect with your breath, your body, doing what feels best for you." Branch recalled doing tree poses during her yoga teacher training and her teacher reminding her trees don't stand still. They move. "You don't have to be this perfectly still tree," she said. "Expand your branches. It's OK to fall down and play in the poses."

When It's Time to Try Tinkering

Have you ever found yourself facing a big dilemma or decision in your life, and you have no idea how to go about solving it? Try tinkering. The tactile experience of working with our hands can help us work through other things going on in our lives.

"Tinker means playing around with things, ideas, and trying out something to see what happens," Dr. Alan Castel, a professor of cognitive psychology at the University of California, Los Angeles, who studies metacognition and aging, wrote for *Psychology Today*. "Often, tinkering is done with some goal in mind, but also sometimes just for the sheer pleasure of trying something out to see what happens."

For some of us, the idea of sitting still, meditating, doing yoga, or even going for a walk doesn't seem to be what we need when we're trying to work through something. When I mentioned to DuShaun Branch, my friend who teaches yoga and whom you were introduced to in the yoga section, how much I love hitting a boxing bag when I am stressed out and need to work through some stuff, she wasn't surprised. She said my personality is such that I need to be actively doing something in order to calm down.

Brian Carberry, an editor based in Atlanta, Georgia, is the same way. "For me, the best way to calm down is to be active," he told me. "I find when I'm sitting still is when my brain gets active, but if I'm physically doing something, my brain is more likely to focus on that activity."

Carberry tries to go on at least one long hike a month, but he also tries to do more things with his hands. "I've crafted DIY photo coasters using backsplash tile and bought a soy wax candle kit, a case of mason jars, and essential oils to create my own candles," he shared. "Both ended up being homemade Christmas gifts for family members this past year."

Many of us tethered to a computer screen most of the day for work purposes know we don't get our best creative ideas at a desk. We need to get out of our typical environment to see ideas or solutions through a different lens. Although it's become a cliché, there is some truth to people coming up with their most creative ideas while showering or working on something completely unrelated. It's like we're giving our brains a mini vacation by letting them focus on something else.

Therein lies the benefits of tinkering.

"In life, we often have problems to figure out, and seeking

the right materials or drawing on past experience (wisdom?) may allow us to understand how the solution can be well within our grasp," added Castel. "Discovery learning consists of a loop of four stages: observation, reflection, abstraction, and experimentation. These stages of discovery learning can be applied in a number of settings, but in order to engage discovery learning, you need to start with some tinkering."

Vanessa McGrady is a Los Angeles–based writer who looks for any opportunity she can to get away from her computer screen. She loves fixing, reusing, and upcycling things because it saves money while keeping trash out of the landfill. It also gives her something to do with her hands and allows her to unplug for a few hours.

When McGrady's neighbor Nancy passed away, she bought an old, dingy dresser from Nancy's son to help him raise money for his mother's services and as a way to keep her wonderful neighbor's memory alive. Once she got it home, she thought she'd bring it back to life with a different paint color. Her hands got busy. "I started to sand it and I realized how beautiful the wood was. The paint was so old and crappy that it just came right off." For McGrady, the benefit of tinkering is that you don't always know how things will turn out, and that's part of the beauty. "I think tinkering gives you an element of delight and surprise, which is good for your brain."

Sometimes, she said, tinkering can be incredibly frustrating, not unlike trying to figure out something that's complicated. And other times, the tinkering will never have an end date, and that's fine too.

"Tinkering can be frustrating, and it's not always going

to be the thing that you want it to be," McGrady admitted. She is happiest when people enjoy what she's made, whether that's soup or a book or something she did in her garden. "It's something I made that's in the world that may even be there after I'm gone," she added.

Castel believes tinkering using our hands can help us work through problems because it also lets us get away from the problem we're currently facing. Even if solutions don't exactly appear while tinkering, letting yourself get lost in thought is part of that "incubation" period, something research shows we need in order to come up with effective solutions.

"Mind wandering, which can be both intentional but often occurs without our awareness, may be a form of tinkering that allows you to first get away from the problem at hand, think of some related and seemingly unrelated thoughts, and then return with a fresh and more informed perspective," Castel added.

—————————— TRY IT ——————————

1. The great thing about tinkering is you don't need an end goal. You just need to start something. Let your hands get busy.

2. If you don't already have an idea of what you want to do or try, McGrady recommends starting by looking around your environment. What do you notice? Is there a pillow with a seam undone? Or a chair that needs to be fixed? Do you have a garbage can out in the open that looks ugly and boring and you're thinking, "Hmm, maybe I could paint that?" "If it's something you look at every day and it bothers you every

single time you look at it, that's a lot of energy leaking out every single day," she said. "So see what's bothering you and go set aside half an hour," she recommended. "If you can sew up that little rip or paint that thing that's so boring and ugly, then you'll basically have solved a problem for yourself. And then you can free your brain to think about other things."

3. If the project you have in mind is bigger, like painting an entire dresser, don't think about the time it'll take to do the whole thing, since that might not be possible. Instead, like other projects in our lives, break the larger project down into smaller action items. Start by simply scraping off the paint, even if it's just one side. Then paint just one drawer at a time.

4. If you're the kind of person who likes to have something to start and finish in one sitting, Carberry's idea of buying a kit or at least the components you need, whether it's to make coasters or candles, might be a good idea. Think about what you have been wanting to create, and pick up the pieces so you have them on hand for when you need a break.

(17)

Runner's High

When Ken Monarrez started running in his middle school years, little did he know the practice would become his lifeline. He combined his love of being outside and his competitive nature into a sport where he was able to multitask mentally while challenging himself physically.

When he ran track, his coach would say to him, "Find the shoulder blades of the guy or gal in front of you and lock in on their shoulder blades and just go chase him down." Once you pass that person, you focus your eyes on the next set of shoulder blades. Those shoulder blades, Monarrez told me, were moving targets, and that took the pressure off the race. Sometimes when he was in a race, he'd count from zero to whatever number he could get up to, whether it was steps or breaths. All these mind games helped relax him when he was competing, and now, in his forties, he uses a variation of these techniques daily as a runner.

While he appreciates what running brings to his life, it wasn't until he trained for his first marathon in 2008 that he first experienced what's known as a "runner's high."

"You're not thinking about anything else," he said. "You're thinking about how good you feel."

Once you feel that runner's high, he said, you want to feel it again. He doesn't care if it takes three miles or twenty miles.

"It's a little bit of stress but a lot calmer," he said, laughing. As he's gotten older and is battling cancer, he admits it's harder to feel that high. "These days, it's more like chasing the devil away."

Despite the hardships Monarrez has had to deal with, he can always count on running to help pull him through. Even when he was going through cancer recovery and when he couldn't physically run, the *idea* that he'd get the chance to run again was the mental gymnastics he needed to do to get him to the other side of treatments. He wanted to feel his feet hit the ground. He wanted to feel his heart pumping.

"Every Monday morning, at 8:00 a.m., this quote from *Born to Run* pops up on my telephone screen. 'Beyond the very extreme of fatigue and distress, we may find amounts of ease and power we never dreamed ourselves to own; sources of strength never taxed at all because we never push through the obstruction.'"

This quote is how he centers himself for the day. Today might be tough or today might not be tough, he added, but you need to persevere and push through it, and that's the same philosophy he carries through as a runner.

When he needs to work through something or clear his head, a thirty-minute hard run will help. "I know if I've had a bad day at work, and I can't get my brain to function and get back in line, I'll run for thirty minutes," he explained. "Like just hammer it down and go and run hard. And I come back with a clear mind and a clear heart."

This clearing or calming of the mind and body is a common thread among runners and one of the reasons the practice has thousands of devotees pounding the pavement daily. In his book *Running Is My Therapy*, author Scott Douglas shared how running changed his life and interviewed experts to explain why running can make a difference not only for those suffering from depression or anxiety but also for those who simply want to build better habits and enjoy living a happier life.

Cindy Kuzma is a runner, journalist, podcaster, and author of several books on running, including *Breakthrough Women's Running: Dream Big and Train Smart* and *Rebound: Train Your Mind to Bounce Back Stronger from Sports Injuries*. She counts on running to help calm her mind and body and considers breathing to be a big part of that experience.

"Most of the time, I don't listen to podcasts or music when I'm running," Kuzma explained. "Instead, I sync my footsteps to my inhalations and exhalations, with the exact pattern depending on the pace (four steps in, four out, for an easy run; two in, two out for a hard, fast workout). I then count them in sets that also depend on the effort level."

As an example, for an easy run, each eight-count breath is one, and she tries to stay focused enough to count up to one thousand. For a hard workout, she counts ten sets of ten, then starts over again. "It truly keeps me in the present moment and focused on what I am doing right then, letting other stressors and distractions fade away," she added. "It's also just an incredible way to bring my body back to equilibrium. If I'm angry or aggravated, a harder run can release some of that pent-up tension, leaving me calmer. If I'm sad, an easy long run where I'm admiring the beauty of the lakefront and the sounds of the birds lifts my spirits—and leaves me feeling accomplished. There's also a huge sense of community in running. I can go on the lakefront trail and see other people I know or other people who love running like I do, and I instantly feel calmer and more connected."

Among the experts Douglas references is Panteleimon Ekkekakis, PhD, a researcher and professor of exercise physiology at Iowa State University, who notes regular running produces the same two changes that are thought to be responsible for the effectiveness of modern antidepressants: increased levels of the neurotransmitters serotonin and norepinephrine, and neurogenesis—the creation of new brain cells.

Ekkekakis also notes that "after a run, there is a drop in blood pressure, and your heart rate and systolic blood pressure don't increase in response to typical emotional stressors in the way they do when you haven't worked out."

People often talk about going for a run to "clear their head," and Douglas talks about this in his book too. "When people talk about clearing their mind with a good run, they can mean getting rid of thoughts that have bedraggled them for the last however many hours. That can happen because of distraction ('gosh, look at the pretty flowers') or focus ('the most important thing in the world right now is that I run this fifth eight-hundred-meter repeat as fast as the first four')."

Kuzma understands running can feel hard and anxiety-inducing at first, but keep at it and there's a magic transformation. "Sometime around a month or so, if you're running three times a week, your body starts to get the hang of it, and you realize there is such fluidity in the movement," she added. "I will never be a fast runner with a beautiful stride, but I still see it as a powerful way to both connect to the ground under my feet and explore the world around me. And solve any conundrums I have, including writer's block. I can stare at the screen for hours, stuck, but when I leave the computer and hit the road, words rearrange themselves in my brain to form the sentences that were escaping me."

In some cases, clearing the mind isn't about getting rid of thoughts but actually processing them. Sometimes it's just about appreciating what you have going well in your life.

"When I'm in a really good place and my head's clear, I could run for days," Monarrez said. "And I will tell you, I don't have three thoughts that go through my head." He's not paying attention to the trees or smelling the earth around him. He's just soaking in the feeling of being in a good place. Except when he's hungry. "If I'm hungry, I tend to smell everything," he said with a laugh. "Then I can tell you that there's, like, ten restaurants within six blocks from where I am."

─────────── TRY IT ───────────

1 Even if you don't have plans to run a marathon, getting properly fitted running shoes will help reduce the risk of injury to your feet, ankles, or legs. Most specialized running stores have the ability to fit you (for free), and it usually requires simply testing different types of running shoes on a specialized treadmill that records where your foot lands first. A properly fitted shoe will feel snug enough in the heel and mid foot with space for your toes to wiggle but also support your arches if you tend to pronate or supinate when your feet touch the ground. Supination is when your body weight leans toward the outside of your foot, while walking or running with pronation means your weight tends to be more on the inside of your foot.

2 If you're an absolute beginner, start slowly, Kuzma advises. Many beginners choose a program like Couch to 5K because it's an accessible way for a beginner to log some miles by going out just a few times a week. There is an official Couch to 5K program (paid) via a training app, and there are other versions of it in both written and app form (several of which are free). All follow a similar format designed to get you ready to run a 5K race in nine weeks. Kuzma also recommends trying to stick to it, even if you sometimes struggle (and you will). "Some types of movement feel good almost from the first moment," she said. "Because running is high-intensity and high-impact, it does feel a bit uncomfortable as your body adjusts."

3 If you're the kind of person who loves being part of a team or you want accountability or motivation from others, almost every city or neighborhood has a running group you can join. Some running shops host weekly runs on the weekends too. Ask your neighbors or friends if they know of anyone looking for a running partner or groups that meet regularly. Monarrez has what he calls his "running family," who have helped him when he's needed support, encouragement, or affirmation. Find your family or group to create your own informal team and cheer each other on, especially on days when you might find your motivation lacking.

4 If you're the kind of person who loves meeting goals, sign up for a 5K. It's a short enough run that you can train for it within a few months but also long enough to appreciate the progress you're making over time.

5 Enjoy your time outside. I don't know many runners who enjoy running on a treadmill but consider it a necessary evil if they can't get their run outdoors. But if you're lucky enough to be able to run outside, take advantage of the fresh air, and see the seasons change.

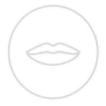

Taste

I think healthy eating overall is taking in something that fulfills you wholly and holistically. It doesn't mean that it has to be "healthy" in terms of whole foods and diets or whatnot, but something that can fulfill you inwardly too. Food is such an instrumental tool in people being able to feel whole.

MOONLYNN TSAI

cofounder of Heart of Dinner, New York City

(18)

Slow Down for Slow Food

Mahatma Gandhi once said, "The best way to find yourself is to lose yourself in the service of others."

Being part of a community can look different to each of us, but there is no mistaking that being part of something that gives us purpose can be so good for our bodies and minds. At its core, community is about connection, and when we feel connected to others, we also feel wanted, loved, and appreciated.

The slow food movement isn't necessarily just about food or making food slowly. It's about connection. It's connection to the food we eat by being mindful of what we're consuming, it's connection by thinking of those who grow our food, and it's connecting with others.

"Slow food brings together the joy of food with food justice," Anna Mulé, executive director of Slow Food USA, told me. "Slow food is about slowing down and a different philosophy of life. It's about not seeing food as a commodity but seeing it in relationships and in connection with many other beings and the earth."

Mulé encourages people to really think about food in connection to our neighbors, whether those neighbors are next door or around the world. Food connects us, after all. There is no escaping the kinship we feel when we prepare a dish for someone or share a meal with friends and family. There is also the element of how the food came to us.

Social connections matter. According to one study, social connection is a pillar of lifestyle medicine: "Humans are wired to connect, and this connection affects our health."

Social support and feeling connected are not only important for people to maintain a healthy body since they help with controlling blood sugar, improving cancer survival, and decreasing cardiovascular mortality, but the authors of the study note they also help decrease depressive symptoms, mitigate post-traumatic stress disorder symptoms, and improve overall mental health. As one would expect and is noted in the study, the opposite of connection—social isolation—has a negative effect on health and can increase depressive symptoms as well as mortality.

Connection Is Medicine

What's great about connecting around food is that food is part of our lives every day. Food is rooted in history and rituals. There is great emphasis among some people that revolves around growing food, making meals from scratch, or preserving a harvest for the next season. Slow Food (capital letters) is a way of life for many. What the Slow Food movement does is connect our interest in food with others and takes it a step further by connecting us with the makers.

In fact, this connection to food and the people who grow our food is an integral part of the Slow Food movement and one that chapters around the country and the world try to develop for their members.

Brekke Bounds is a board member of Slow Food Chicago. When asked the benefits of slow food and how it can help people make stronger connections with each other and the world around us, she finds it's best to let the food speak for itself initially. Then, if people really want to make those connections, she asks them to recall a time when they gathered around food—any type of food will work—with those they cared about, had a good time, and lingered.

For Bounds, slow food isn't always about what we're eating. Slow food is a lifestyle.

"Lingering and connecting over food can and is part of it—and I think it is an easy way to draw attention to a time where many folks can genuinely see benefits," Bounds told me. "They can remember the joy, ease, fun of a moment around food—even if they have been few and far between. If they can extrapolate that to even a couple meals a month, I think they can begin to see how slow food can have benefits to both body and mind."

Bounds admits she tries to live her life as a testament to how caring and giving attention to your food can be a benefit to you. She has seen people around her invest more attention in their food and the ways in which food is produced, and she's always willing to answer any questions and ready to share how easy it is for most people to find room for some slow food in their life.

"Truthfully, I think that many elements of slow food can fit into nearly *any* life with a little bit of intention," she added, noting that she feels thinking about any food with intention can be considered slow food.

─────────────── TRY IT ───────────────

1. There are several ways we can adopt a slow food lifestyle or support the Slow Food movement. For those who are slow food curious, Bounds and Mulé both recommend starting with what moves you first. Is it how food is grown, the preparation of food, the whole conviviality and fellowship around food, food justice, or supporting farmers?

2. Rather than feeling like you have to tackle everything at once, start with one item you really love, whether that's wine, honey, bread, or coffee. Then really look with intentionality into that food chain and try to understand the people behind that product. "Who are the people? What are their issues? How can we be more connected on those issues? That will open a door to these broader conversations that are happening right now," Mulé said.

3. Bounds likes to recommend easy and quick additions to life that can act as a bridge to a slow food lifestyle. "A moment of gratitude before or after a meal that acknowledges the work

of the people who get that food to our plates and the energy that the food will give to us, growing one or two fresh herbs in a small garden or window box, a family walk around a farmers' market or local farm stand and the purchase and eating of just one item (or more as time and money applies)— bonus points for a short conversation with the farmer who grew that food!" Bounds said. "And even if someone never moves beyond one of these items, I would still say they are participating in slow food."

④ Another way to look at adopting a slow food lifestyle or supporting the Slow Food movement is to consider the process like a big "choose your own adventure," according to Bounds. Choosing one of the easy and quick recommendations as a starting point will lead you to more questions or encourage you to learn more about a particular food or how it's farmed, for example. "Your moment of gratitude can turn into research about activism around farm labor or animal rights—or even just the re-creation of an old family recipe that you remember and love," Bounds noted. "Your herb garden can turn into a larger garden or participation in a community garden, or maybe you help start a school garden in your neighborhood. Your trip to the farmers' market can become weekly and you can build friendships with your local farmers, or maybe you start volunteering regularly at the farm to learn more."

⑤ If connecting around food and meeting people appeals to you too, Mulé and Bounds encourage people to get more involved in the Slow Food movement by finding their closest chapter or starting their own. One cannot underestimate the power of connections, and chapters often come together to organize meals. Sometimes those meals have a social justice bent to them to learn about different cultures or different people's views. Sometimes the chapters are more involved in issues such as food access. Whatever the purpose of the gatherings, Slow Food is an organizing tool for people to rally around the community.

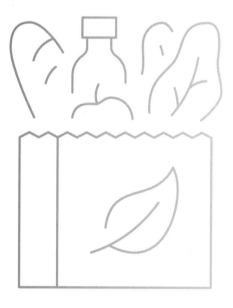

Mood and Food

When I'm stressed, I crave chocolate—like ransacking the pantry for *anything* chocolate. Or bread when I want some comfort food. In the morning, I cannot wait to wrap my hands around my warm cup of coffee and slowly sip it so that morning fog in my head clears and I feel awake and happy.

Could the food we eat have an effect on our mood or vice versa?

The relationship we have with food can and does affect how we feel, and researchers have been studying how food affects our mood and temperament since medieval times. Quince, dates, and elderberries were used as mood enhancers, lettuce and chicory as tranquilizers, and apples, pomegranates, beef, and eggs as erotic stimulants.

Beef as an erotic stimulant? Interesting.

So why exactly do some foods make us sleepy or tired while others get us revved up?

Research continues to shed light on how certain foods change brain structure, chemistry, and physiology, which in turn affect our mood and performance. More specifically, studies suggest that foods directly influencing brain neurotransmitter systems have the greatest effects on mood, at least temporarily. In turn, mood can also influence our food choices, and expectations on the effects of certain foods can influence our perception.

"Serotonin is an important neurotransmitter that the brain produces from tryptophan contained in foods such as clams, oysters, escargots, octopus, squids, banana, pineapple, plum, nuts, milk, turkey, spinach, and eggs," according to an article published in *Dartmouth Undergraduate Journal of Science*. "Functions of serotonin include the regulation of sleep, appetite, and impulse control. Increased serotonin levels are related to mood elevation."

Chocolate is often cited as having a strong effect on mood, and I'm not alone in appreciating how it makes me feel when I eat it. I've had friends compare enjoying a slice of chocolate cake to smoking a cigarette or drinking a cup of coffee. People have chocolate when they're happy or feeling depressed.

"Chocolate contains a number of psychoactive chemicals such as anandamines which stimulate the brain in the same way as cannabis does, tyramine and phenylethylamine which have similar effects as amphetamine, and theobromine and caffeine which act as stimulants," according to research. But it turns out these substances are present in chocolate in very low concentrations. They're not enough to induce an antidepressant effect. What's likely at play is the taste of chocolate in our mouth that is responsible for both our craving and its ability to serve as a mood enhancer.

Caffeine, on the other hand, often consumed as coffee or tea, is the most commonly used legal psychoactive substance in the world. Roughly 80 percent of adult Americans drink coffee daily.

For many of us, the effects of caffeine on our nervous systems are welcomed and include the following:

* Mood changes
* Behavioral changes
* Changes in awareness
* Altered thoughts
* Changes in how we feel

Psychoactive drugs can operate as depressants or stimulants, and how our bodies react to them will differ by person. Caffeine, for example, is considered a stimulant, and stimulants can increase energy, alertness, and wakefulness. For some, caffeine makes them feel jittery and anxious. Alcohol is considered a depressant. While it can calm the brain, cause sleepiness, and make some people feel more relaxed, others experience nightmares, anxiety, and aggression.

Coffee wakes me up, and I enjoy drinking it every morning, but after a certain number of cups, I can feel jittery, so that's my cue to stop drinking it. On the other hand, alcohol really relaxes me but makes me tired, so I tend to have a drink sporadically.

When We Eat and Drink Matters Too

Interestingly, how we feel doesn't stop at what we eat or drink. When we eat or drink can be just as critical to how we show up or what feelings we experience.

I was never a morning person, but since getting married to someone who is, I've slowly adjusted my sleep patterns to mimic my husband's. As I've gotten older, I tend to prioritize my sleep too, so I go to bed earlier. What has happened as a result is what I eat and drink in the morning and early afternoon affects my mood and productivity. Where I used to get by without eating breakfast and relying on coffee, that no longer works. I'll get moody and tired and feel more anxious.

There is a reason for this that goes beyond what each of us eats, and much of it depends "on the time of day, the type and macronutrient composition of food, the amount of food consumed, and the age and dietary history of the subject."

In one study, it was reported that the food choices of "early birds," who feel most productive during the first part of the day, become particularly important during lunch and throughout the afternoon, while "night owls" feel most energetic later in the day and should pay attention to their breakfast choices as they can increase or decrease energy levels and influence cognitive functioning.

Identifying what foods make us feel good can help us carry on our days in a way that serves us. And if something doesn't taste good or makes us feel lousy, that's a good reason to consider alternatives.

——————————— TRY IT ———————————

1. Keep a food journal and note how you feel before, during, and after you eat or drink something. It took me years to realize coffee made me anxious if I drank it after noon. I still drink way more coffee than I should, but I've learned what energizes me and when to stop.

2. Food sensitivities and allergies are real. Some ingredients or foods can give you headaches, for example. Others might make you irritable or uncomfortable. Keeping a food journal might help identify those triggers so you can avoid those foods or ingredients.

3. Take time to enjoy what you're eating. This might sound obvious, but we're often living in a fast-paced world with overscheduled days. Eat a well-balanced diet, stay away from processed foods, and don't skip meals. Make food a pleasure to eat, not something to check off on your never-ending list of things to do.

4. Another thing I've tried to do more regularly is plan ahead. When life gets too busy (and life will *always* get in the way), it's helpful to have a plan B. Meal plan and prep, for example, on the weekends, and freeze a few meals for those days when you can't properly prepare a healthy meal. You won't stress or feel anxious about figuring out what to eat or need to rely on unhealthy food that doesn't even taste good.

Culinary Therapy

For most of us, cooking needs to happen so we can eat and stay alive. It's often a daily practice, and unlike some activities, cooking involves all our senses. What if we approached cooking as a form of daily meditation?

"Think of the last time you cooked. Were you rushed, calm, fluid, or scrambled?" Heather L. Nickrand, MA, LPC, NCC, a hospice regional bereavement and volunteer manager with AMITA Health, asked me. "Many times, how we feel is more true in how we cook."

While Nickrand mostly works with clients who recently lost a close family member or friend and uses culinary therapy in her practice, she recognizes the impact food and mindful cooking can have on our health and well-being.

"We are truly honest and vulnerable in our cooking," Nickrand added. "Exploring movement therapy is fascinating in cooking. The self-awareness and honesty is in the movements. This allows us to explore self-care strategies and be mindful of our needs."

Cooking and baking are activities that are considered behavioral activation by therapists, according to a *Wall Street Journal* article on how cooking can help treat depression and anxiety. "The goal of culinary therapy is to alleviate depression by boosting positive activity," Jeanne Whalen, the author of the article, said. "As a result, goal-oriented behavior increases, and procrastination and passivity are curbed."

There are a few things at play when people embark on cooking as an activity, either as an occasional event or a daily ritual. For one thing, it requires some focus to cook something, and that helps tune out other things swirling in your mind. In a study published in the *Journal of Happiness Studies*, young adults who engaged in "maker activities" such as cooking, baking, or gardening showed positive subjective well-being. Among the most important reasons they said they were engaging in these types of activities were mood repair, socializing with friends, and the ability to "stay present- focused."

Even avid cooks find the act of preparing a meal therapeutic. "Preparing a meal is unlike anything else I do in the course of a day," said food writer Ellen Kanner in an article for *Psychology Today* on how kitchen therapy can be beneficial for mental well-being. "It's a nourishing, centering act that gets me to slow down and focus."

All five of our senses, especially taste, are engaged fully when cooking, and that contributes to our overall health and well-being.

——————————— TRY IT ———————————

Does this sound like you? You finish your day and you're wired. You need to prepare dinner, but you don't know what to make because your head is still reeling from the day's events, whether they were exciting or horrible.

If your mind is scrambled and busy thinking about what happened during the day or what happened yesterday or what might happen tomorrow, it'll be hard to focus on the task at hand or to be present.

So how can you use cooking to help you calm your body and mind?

First, take a deep breath before you even walk into your kitchen or as soon as you arrive. You know you're going to be doing some prep work and will be in the kitchen for a specific amount of time, so make a deal with yourself that during that time, you're going to focus on the task of preparing and cooking this meal, and you'll return to whatever needs your attention later.

As you go through your tasks, consider naming your actions. "I'm adding water into the pot. I'm cutting this vegetable. I'm placing the dish into the oven."

Allow yourself to notice each of your senses as you're deciding what to make and how you prepare your dish.

* How do the ingredients smell as you prepare your meal? Are you inhaling their aroma and taking a deep breath as you're working?

✳ How does the vegetable feel in your hands, or what do you feel when you're stirring the pot? Is it smooth to the touch or coarse?

✳ Are you tasting your dish as you're working? Acknowledge the taste. Is it sweet, salty, tangy? Stay in the moment and be present. What might your dish need?

✳ As you're working, really listen. Can you identify any patterns, whether it's your knife cutting a vegetable or the sound of sauce simmering in the pot?

✳ How is your dish shaping up? Take a moment to admire your process. What colors are in your dish? Can you make it more colorful? "Incorporating colors in your food improves mental wellness!" Nickrand shared.

✳ Find a cooking partner. Remember, not all meals need to be prepared solo. If you can prepare your meal with someone else or a community of people even on some days of the week or month, see if that activity might be good for you.

(21)

Tea (or Coffee) Time

For many of us, drinking our first cup of coffee or tea in the morning is about more than just a hot drink to get us going. It's a ritual, an experience, a moment of tranquility. It's deeply satisfying and comforting.

It's also pretty calming, and there are several reasons we crave those first few caffeinated sips in the morning or look forward to our tea break in the afternoon.

Jennifer Billock, an author of several books and a certified tea specialist, loves the ritual of preparing her loose-leaf tea. "You weigh out the [loose-leaf] tea and you heat the water to a certain temperature based on what kind of tea you're having," she told me. "There's a science to it, there's a ritual to it, and it becomes something calming for me to do in the morning."

That calming effect goes beyond the preparation for Billock. She takes in the whole experience, including holding a warm mug and enjoying the feeling she gets from both the smell of the tea and having the steam in her face.

To hear Billock talk about tea is to hear her speak as if it's a form of meditation. "I think it's more of a mental moment," she added. "To kind of calm down and recognize what's going on in your day and what's going on in your life and having something warm to drink to help you through that."

Most of us think teas, especially green and black teas, are a rich source of flavonoids, and that's the reason tea helps calm our nerves when we drink it. While research continues to prove that flavonoids—natural polyphenol-like compounds found commonly in plants, fruits, vegetables, and medicinal herbs—might have potential therapeutic effects for the treatment of brain-associated disorders, including anxiety and depression, there might be something else at play when it comes to drinking green tea: the L-theanine amino acid.

L-theanine is a unique nonprotein amino acid found in green tea. Some studies show that increasing intake of theanine can significantly reduce symptoms of anxiety, such as a racing heartbeat.

Does that mean you have to swap your favorite black tea for green tea? Nope. Daily cups of any kind of tea can help you recover more quickly from the stresses of everyday life, according to Andrew Steptoe, professor at the UCL Department of Epidemiology and Health and lead author of a study published in the journal *Psychopharmacology*.

He and his coauthors set out to see whether the reason people feel this way is due to the relaxing situations in which they're enjoying their tea or the biological ingredients of tea.

One group in this study was given a fruit-flavored caffeinated tea mixture made up of the constituents of an average cup of black tea. The other group was given a caffeinated placebo identical in taste but devoid of the active tea ingredients.

The verdict? The study suggests that drinking black tea may speed up our recovery from the daily stresses in life based on the ingredients of tea, according to Steptoe. "Although it does not appear to reduce the actual levels of stress we experience, tea does seem to have a greater effect in bringing stress hormone levels back to normal," he noted. While the study was not able to determine which of the ingredients were responsible for these effects on stress recovery and relaxation, he added that ingredients in tea such as catechins, polyphenols, flavonoids, and amino acids have been found to have effects on the brain's neurotransmitters.

It's important to note here that both tea and coffee contain caffeine, and caffeine is a drug because it stimulates the central nervous system. This is why we rely on our morning cup of joe for that energy boost and why drinking it improves our mood. It makes us more alert and enhances our concentration.

While consuming drinks with caffeine can be beneficial, moderation is key.

"In large doses, caffeine has been associated with anxiety, restlessness, and difficulty sleeping," Lisa Wartenberg, MFA, RD, LD, wrote for *Healthline*. "In addition, some studies suggest that drinking it regularly, even in moderate amounts, can cause chronic headaches and migraines."

Does this mean we have to give up our caffeinated drinks?

Not at all. I, for one, look forward to my morning coffee. I always enjoy it black.

For me, it's more than just the jolt in the morning, although that's a nice perk. Like how Billock experiences her tea, I'm drawn to the way the coffee smells when it's brewing. The anticipation is a big part of my morning ritual. As it brews, I grab my pen and journal. Once the coffee is ready, I pour some into my favorite mug—a hand-thrown pottery mug I bought one summer while I was traveling with my family since it's a nice reminder of a fun trip. Holding it in my hands, wrapping my fingers around the mug, makes me happy. The coffee is hot, so my hands warm pretty quickly. My day honestly doesn't begin until I take that first sip. And it's a sip I savor because it tastes so good and so comforting.

It's hard to convince a non–coffee or tea drinker to start their own ritual because people seem to have strong opinions about them. Kind of like if you're a cat person or a dog person, you either love coffee or hate it. You either drink tea or you don't. If you're a hard-core coffee drinker and willing to give tea a chance, Billock encourages coffee friends to try a glass of Lapsang souchong tea because she feels it's the most similar to coffee. But if you're willing to try something new, here are some tips to get you started on your own journey.

——————————————— TRY IT ———————————————

1 There are thousands of varieties of tea but only six categories: black, oolong, green, white, yellow, and pu'erh. Just like coffee, no teas are the same, and you really need to try different types to get a sense of what you like and what you don't.

2   On the coffee side, there are four different types of coffee beans: arabica, robusta, liberica, and excelsa. You'll most likely find coffee or drinks made from arabica and robusta as they're the most popular and commonly found.

3   Rather than buying larger containers of tea leaves or coffee beans, head to a local coffee shop when it's not busy, and take your time looking over the menu of offerings. Ask the barista about the types of coffees they sell. Depending on the coffee shop and how busy they are, many are more than happy to talk about their drinks. Also, many times shops will have sample packs or smaller containers so customers can try tasting a variety of teas or coffees before investing in larger packets.

4   If you have a friend who loves a particular type of coffee or tea, ask for their recommendations. I love the taste of coconut, for example, so I usually gravitate toward those flavor profiles even in my coffee or tea. I also love the taste of rose or hibiscus, so I'll often try tea or coffee with those flavors. They're not always a win, but I don't regret trying them. I found one of my favorite go-to coffees that way. Since I tend to try a lot of coffee and tea, I have a stash at home at the ready when guests come over. Your friends might even invite you over to drink some of their own favorites.

5   Enjoy the whole experience, and don't be afraid to taste something new. I love chocolate, but I've not found a coffee or tea to brew at home that has that chocolate flavoring I love. I'll order a mocha or latte at a coffee shop instead. I wasn't

expecting to like coconut in my coffee, though, and now I have that as my go-to coffee at home.

6 Create a ritual around the experience. Use a mug you really love. Carve out time in your day to drink your tea or coffee in silence or as a little break.

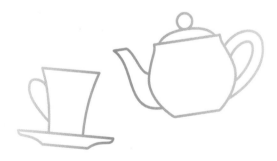

22

Spice It Up

When most of us think of herbs and spices, we think of how they affect our taste buds, not necessarily our minds. But as is the case with many foods and drinks, herbs and spices often evoke memories and have healing properties that go beyond flavoring a dish.

According to Kaumudi Marathé, chef/writer and founder of Un-Curry (un-curry.com), spices and herbs have nutritional benefits that help the body on many fronts, be it reducing bad cholesterol (coriander seed), making proteins more easily digestible (asafetida), reducing inflammation (turmeric), lowering blood sugar (cinnamon), promoting lactation (fenugreek seed), improving digestion (ginger), adding iron to the system (cumin, curry leaves), or easing perimenopausal symptoms (cilantro, coriander seed, wild asparagus). Marathé aims to shatter the myth of stereotypical

Indian cuisine by serving up regional dishes that reflect the diversity and history of an ancient land through Un-Curry, which offers cooking classes, pop-up restaurant opportunities, and catering services. At Un-Curry, she blends seasonal, organic, California ingredients with Indian spices, culinary techniques, and Ayurvedic philosophy.

"To my mind, the most important thing about spices and herbs is the fact that they transform ingredients that might otherwise be boring or even unpleasant to eat, like cabbage or bitter melon, into delectable bites and the beautiful food memories they evoke," Marathé told me.

Herbs and spices do elevate our foods, and they've been used for centuries for culinary and medicinal purposes. According to one study, "there is now ample evidence that spices and herbs possess antioxidant, anti-inflammatory, anti-tumorigenic, anticarcinogenic, and glucose- and cholesterol-lowering activities as well as properties that affect cognition and mood."

Marathé recognizes the power these ingredients have on our bodies and minds. When she smells powdered coriander and cumin seeds, she is immediately transported to her paternal grandparents' home in Pune, a city in the western Indian state of Maharashtra, where her grandmother sautéed cabbage with them. Freshly minced cilantro as a garnish on lentils or on an Indian salad fills her nostrils with its fragrance, making her hungry, and satisfies her with every coconut-y bite.

"Indeed, even before a meal is ready to eat, just smelling herbs and spices while the food is cooking makes you salivate and gets your digestive juices going," she added. "Then when you start eating, your body is ready to receive the nutrition. Of course, you taste the spices and herbs while you eat and enjoy their aroma, crunch, texture, and flavor."

As many of us who love Indian cuisine know, Indians use a lot of spices and a few herbs (cilantro, mint, bay leaf, and curry leaves) in their cooking, and Marathé studied these so she could understand what they bring to Indian food. She wrote about them in *The Essential Marathi Cookbook* because, for the most part, according to Marathé, Indian food writers and cooks of the past had not consciously talked about the health benefits of spices and herbs, even if they inherently understood they were good for you.

"Mothers, fathers, grandmothers would say things like, 'black pepper is good for you,' but I wanted to move beyond that ambiguity and document the benefits in some way for a younger generation that was distanced from family and cooks who knew traditional ways deeply," she said.

As the study reported, many herbs and spices have positive health properties to help stave off disease. Marathé agrees and notes that all the spices and herbs used in regional Indian food have medicinal and nutritional benefits, whether it is the anti-inflammatory, antiseptic, antioxidant qualities of turmeric, the ability of coriander seed and cinnamon to help reduce cholesterol, or the iron content of cumin and curry leaves. "These were discovered over centuries of cooking with these spices and learning which ingredients they best paired with," she said. "In India, there was a need for cooling the body, obtaining minerals and fiber that might be unavailable or scarce in the hot months, and for preserving ingredients in the days before refrigeration. In France, for instance, people made herbes de Provence to preserve summer herbs. In India, they made spice blends like garam masala (NO curry powder!) annually. They also pickled fruit and vegetables with spices and often oil to preserve them."

Experimentation, she added, is what led to discoveries about what worked and what didn't and what spices complemented each other and worked well for different ingredients and seasons.

For all the health and wellness benefits herbs and spices afford us, Marathé doesn't use them in the sense of well-being. Instead, she draws her comfort from being in the kitchen and different aspects of cooking.

"I enjoy the soothing repetitive action of cutting vegetables, the round motion of stirring cake batter, or the robustness of making pasta sauce," Marathé noted. "I enjoy the aromas I smell as I cut, chop, and blend. Most of all, I think I enjoy the aromatic activity of making an Indian spice-and-oil seasoning. When those black mustard seeds pop in the hot oil and smell like freshly popped corn, I feel like I've come home."

TRY IT

For those who want to incorporate more herbs and spices into their lives, Marathé has some specific recommendations and suggestions.

1 India has a unique way of using spices as hot oil and spice seasoning, which she shares in her cooking classes. "The oil/ghee and heat release the flavors and goodness of spices into

food," she said. "People here don't necessarily know about this or understand the way to use spices. For instance, many people don't know that turmeric has to be heated before it is consumed because heat slows down its progress through the body, making it more bioavailable to us. That's why all those turmeric root smoothies don't do very much! People also don't know about brown/black mustard seeds. They come from the same plant as yellow mustard but are more commonly used in Indian cooking."

2 Second, she tells her students they don't have to go out and invest in a spice cupboard full of Indian spices and try cooking complicated Indian meals. "Go easy on yourself," she advised. She recommends learning the basic seasoning techniques and starting with the spices you have at home. Just try making one dish with a spice you have on hand. If you have cumin seed, for instance, make an oil seasoning with it, and sauté some broccoli florets in the seasoned oil. "That humdrum broccoli will take on new life," she said. "If you have turmeric, rub it on pieces of salmon with some salt and panfry them. A squeeze of lemon and you've got an amazing fish course."

3 Be willing to experiment. While some people rely on "safe" herbs and spices like salt or basil or crushed pepper, Marathé recommends using a spice unfamiliar to you with an ingredient that is familiar, so it is not altogether strange to eat. "Bring spinach alive by sautéing it with garlic, mustard seed, turmeric, and asafetida. You need to learn the seasoning technique though," Marathé said. "Sprinkle powdered cumin over chopped tomato and onion for an out-of-this-world fragrant salad."

④ Finally, consider the age of your herbs and spices and where you store them. Marathé recommends never using spice powders that are over three months old or that look pale brown. "They have lost their aroma and add no flavor to food," she said. "Grind your own spice powders fresh, with a mortar and pestle or a coffee grinder reserved for spices. Grind enough for a couple of weeks and store in an airtight jar."

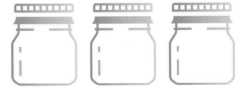

23

Let Food Be Thy Medicine

It might have been 400 BC when Greek physician Hippocrates, considered to be the founder of modern medicine, said, "Let food be thy medicine and let medicine be thy food," but the sentiment still rings true today.

Researchers in the emerging field of nutritional psychiatry are finding a notable link between what you eat and what you feel, particularly when it comes to managing depression and anxiety.

Dr. Eva Selhub describes nutritional psychiatry as your brain on food and likens the brain to an expensive car. "Like an expensive car, your brain functions best when it gets only premium fuel," Selhub wrote for Harvard Health Publishing. "Eating high-quality foods that contain lots of vitamins, minerals, and antioxidants nourishes the brain and protects it from oxidative stress—the 'waste' (free radicals) produced when the body uses oxygen, which can damage cells."

Continuing with the expensive car analogy, your brain can become damaged if you fuel it with anything other than premium fuel. When "lowgrade" fuel, such as processed or refined foods, reaches the brain, it has little ability to get rid of the toxins.

"Diets high in refined sugars, for example, are harmful to the brain," Selhub wrote. "In addition to worsening your body's regulation of insulin, they also promote inflammation and oxidative stress. Multiple studies have found a correlation between a diet high in refined sugars and impaired brain function—and even a worsening of symptoms of mood disorders, such as depression."

About 95 percent of serotonin—a neurotransmitter that helps regulate sleep and appetite, mediate moods, and inhibit pain—is produced in the gastrointestinal tract, and how the body rids itself of toxins is important.

The "gut-brain axis," as registered dietitian and nutritionist Wesley Delbridge explains it, ties our digestive systems to how we feel.

"We're realizing our gut talks to our brain and it can have huge effects on our mood and the emotions we experience," Delbridge said. "If your gut is happy, then you're going to be more happy."

How do we make our gut happy? By making sure our digestive systems get more of the "good" bacteria so they can protect the lining of our intestines and ensure they provide a strong barrier against toxins and "bad" bacteria. Those good bacteria also limit inflammation, improve how well we absorb nutrients from our food, and activate neural pathways that travel directly between the gut and the brain.

While there are some foods that generally are good for our bodies and minds, it's important to recognize that we're all unique, so what helps one person might not have the same effect on another person.

Gina Caruso, an integrative nutrition health coach and founder of Caruso Coaching, explained the term *bio-individuality*, which means we're all unique and there's no one-size-fits-all approach to health and nutrition, so she encourages clients to first understand how food affects them. Before we can get to what types of foods help calm us, we must first bring awareness of how the foods we currently eat make us feel without making any changes.

How do we do this? "Just bring an awareness to the foods you're eating now," Caruso recommends. And note how you feel before, during, and after eating those foods. It doesn't need to be a complicated process. Simply keeping a food journal can be the first step to making yourself aware by noting what you eat and how you feel.

As a nutritionist, Caruso makes it a point to add that how our bodies and minds feel around food is more than just the transaction of putting food in our mouths. It's also about thinking about food and the type of food we want to have. Digestion begins once we begin *thinking* of food. Our salivary glands amp up, and our senses become aware. Then the actual practice of eating food comes into play, and Caruso always asks people to bring mindfulness to how they're eating the food.

For example, if a food is traditionally thought of as calming but eaten under stress, it could still cause distress in the body. So rather than just focusing on the food we're consuming, Caruso asks us to consider the environment in which we're eating as well. "Really bring awareness to when one is eating," she said. "If one can actually get away from electronics or other distractions, you can create an uplifted environment, which all contributes to the food having a calming effect, in addition to the actual food."

While each of us is different and our dietary needs vary, there is something to be said about the oft-used comment: we are what we eat. So if we want to influence how our bodies and minds feel, there does seem to be some agreement among experts that whole and plant-based diets rich in vegetables, fruits, unprocessed grains, and fish and seafood and containing only modest amounts of lean meats and dairy are preferable to processed and refined foods and sugars more common in "Western" diets. Many of these unprocessed foods are fermented and therefore act as natural probiotics, according to Selhub.

A meta-analysis suggests that adherence to a "healthful" dietary pattern, comprising higher intakes of fruit and vegetables, fish, and whole grains, is associated with a reduced likelihood of depression in adults.

Another study found that those with depressive symptoms had a "significant reduction" after twelve weeks on a healthy diet. While the study's authors did recognize there are many versions of a "healthful diet" among different countries and cultures, the available evidence from observational studies notes that diets higher in plant foods, such as vegetables, fruits, legumes, and whole grains, and lean proteins, including fish, are associated with a reduced risk for depression, while dietary patterns that include more processed food and sugary products are associated with an increased risk of depression.

The *World Journal of Psychiatry* published a paper listing twelve antidepressant nutrients related to the prevention and treatment of depressive disorders. Those twelve nutrients that have shown to improve one's mood are folate, iron, long-chain omega-3 fatty acids (EPA and DHA), magnesium, potassium, selenium, thiamine, vitamin A, vitamin B6, vitamin B12, vitamin C, and zinc. According to the report, the highest scoring foods were bivalves such as oysters and mussels, various seafoods, and organ meats for animal foods. The highest scoring plant foods were leafy greens, lettuces, peppers, and cruciferous vegetables.

Key nutrients your body receives from eating certain foods can influence the levels of serotonin, while other nutrients can help prevent inflammation so blood circulates well to all your organs.

It's worth noting that what you eat is only part of the equation. The environment in which you eat matters.

Eating with intention cannot be underestimated. "It's connected to that sense of fight or flight," Caruso said. In this case, it's rest and digest. "In order for the body to actually properly digest food, it has to be in a pretty calm state."

To get to a calm state, people need to not be stressed out or distracted. Try to take just ten minutes to walk away from your desk when you eat. Get to a table if you can. Enjoy your meal, and use proper posture.

"These things sound like they're inconsequential, but they're actually quite important for that whole experience of being able to calm oneself down, have proper digestion, and really appreciate the food on one's plate," Caruso added. By taking that time to be present while you're eating, you can enjoy the sense of taste too. Make sure you're chewing your food and appreciating the texture of each bite. If you rush to eat something, not only are you being dismissive of the food, but you're depriving yourself of that wonderful sensory experience of enjoying your food.

"We don't give ourselves enough credit for having the inner wisdom to know what's right or wrong for our bodies," Caruso said. "Our bodies are so intelligent. They provide us with a lot of information if we just bring an awareness and listen."

"People should literally trust their gut," she added, especially as it helps bring awareness to how food is affecting them. Caruso also recommends people take the leap to go see a nutritionist and perhaps get some blood work done. After getting those results, consider working with a certified health coach to help you find what works for you and make some permanent changes in your life.

It's possible to bring some joy around food again, she insists. Food doesn't need to be serious. It can be fun too.

—————————————————— TRY IT ——————————————————

1. If it's hard to get fruit or vegetable servings throughout the day, try to get them in meals you already eat. Add a banana to your breakfast routine and vegetables in sauces or soup with your dinner.

② Another tip is to preplan so when you're tempted to reach for a cookie or candy bar, you can just as easily reach for something healthy. Keep cut-up vegetables and fruits at eye level in the refrigerator so they're the first thing you see when you open it, and you're more likely to grab them when a snack craving hits.

③ Include foods rich in omega-3 fatty acids, such as salmon, in your weekly diet. Dark green leafy vegetables are brain protective. And if you're like me and dislike the taste of some things raw or cooked, experiment! While I don't love raw spinach, I like it cooked in dishes. My friend hates cooked broccoli but loves snacking on it raw.

④ Nuts, seeds, and legumes, such as beans and lentils, are excellent brain foods.

⑤ Dark chocolate contains flavonols and antioxidants in the flavonoid family, which may increase blood flow in arteries, reduce the stickiness of blood platelets, and lower blood pressure.

⑥ Finally, don't forget to engage your senses while eating. Take the time to really taste your food. Feel how your body reacts when you consume certain foods. Inhale the aroma as you prepare your meals or bring your fork to your lips. Add as many colors as possible to your dish so it's pleasantly appealing while healthy for your mind and body.

(24)

Mindful Eating

The secret to mindful eating is focusing on the food you eat and allowing yourself the time to enjoy its texture, color, aroma, and taste. What mindful eating is not is a diet.

Living in a world of being perpetually busy, it's no wonder we rush through eating our meals—if we bother to eat at all. If we forget to eat, our bodies remind us, either through cues in our stomach or headaches or irritability that causes us to snap at people. We then rush again to find sustenance. We drive through a fast-food restaurant or grab a chocolate bar or salty chips from a vending machine, and then we feel sluggish the rest of the day.

We've become so accustomed to multitasking as a way of life that we cannot sit still and just enjoy what we're doing at this moment, and that includes eating a meal.

Stress contributes to mindless eating, which occurs when

we're distracted from what we're eating or eating when we're not hungry. Scarfing down whatever's closest to us because we've forgotten to eat, eating because we're bored, eating while distracted like when watching a show or scrolling through our phone, or eating when we're angry or worried are all examples of mindless eating. Stress is a major contributor to mindless eating.

And unlike other ways to manage stress, eating food is something we all must do to stay alive. Food is easily accessible and legal (unlike drugs or alcohol), which makes it easier to use as a drug or emotional anesthetic.

At the heart of mindless eating are our habits of living on autopilot and stress. Often, it's not hunger that drives it at all.

Elissa Epel, founder and director of the Center for Obesity Assessment, Study, and Treatment at the University of California, San Francisco, has been researching the role of stress in overeating. According to Epel, one of the biggest, most reliable paths to obesity is high stress because it changes our appetite, stimulates overeating, and makes us more insulin-resistant, a factor that elevates blood sugar and can put us at risk for type 2 diabetes.

"Stress affects the same signals as famine does. It turns on the brain pathways that make us crave dense calories—we'll choose high fat, high sweet, or high salt foods," said Epel in an article published in *Greater Good* magazine. "When we have a 'stress brain,' food is even more rewarding."

Mindfulness can help. Mindfulness teaches you to be less reactive to stress and reduce emotional eating.

"Feeling stressed out is a common trigger of mindless

eating, even for the healthiest of eaters," said Dr. Susan Albers, a psychologist at the Cleveland Clinic who specializes in eating issues, weight loss, body image concerns, and mindfulness. In her book *Eating Mindfully*, she shares the story of Linda who, like many of us, needed time to relax from her day so she developed an automatic habit of reaching for food as a way to unwind. Judging by what she chose, she was likely more stressed than hungry. "Food can comfort and soothe because it instantly changes your senses and distracts you," Albers noted. "Sometimes it's easier to eat mindlessly than to deal directly with the source of stress, particularly if it is something like confronting your boss or apologizing to your spouse."

Stress doesn't always cause people to eat poorly. For some, too much stress might have the opposite effect. Instead of resorting to grabbing whatever will soothe, you lose your appetite so you don't feel or notice your hunger.

When you participate in mindful eating, you're choosing to be aware of what you're eating and how much you're eating and appreciate the flavor of your food. "Mindful eating is feeling the food in your stomach and experiencing pleasure—or whatever you feel—from eating it," Albers wrote.

At first blush, this way of eating might seem time-consuming and stressful, yet Albers notes in her book that mindful eating doesn't have to take a lot of time or require radical changes.

In another book Albers wrote, *Eat, Drink, and Be Mindful*, she shared that the first step of mindful eating involves noticing all the senses, tastes, smells, and textures of the food eaten. The second is recognizing repetitive habits, such as eating while multitasking and eating on autopilot without being aware consciously. The third is being aware of what triggers the initiation and cessation of eating.

Mindful eating is not a diet. Rather, it's about focusing on the process of eating, not what is eaten.

—————————————— TRY IT ——————————————

With these tips in mind, here are some ways to practice mindful eating:

1 Slow down. Nutrition experts say that it can take up to twenty minutes before your body realizes it's full. Eat your meal slowly so you can enjoy it, and let your body and mind catch up to your activity.

2 Create a healthy eating environment. Remove distractions and unhealthy foods from your pantry or countertop so you're not tempted to engage in unhealthy habits.

3 Following that idea, turn off the television, or set aside your phone or device in another room so you're not tempted to use them as a form of distraction.

4 Take stock of how you're feeling before resorting to a snack or meal. Ask yourself, "Am I eating because I am hungry, or am I eating because I am [insert your emotion: sad/excited/ nervous]?" Paying attention to your hunger cues can help you determine if you're trying to satisfy a hunger pang or

masking another issue that should be addressed. If you're not actually hungry, try engaging in a different activity instead—like going for a walk, taking a shower, or picking up a book.

5 Record how your body feels when you eat mindlessly versus when you eat mindfully. An example Albers offers in *Eating Mindfully* is when you eat mindlessly, symptoms might include weakness, headaches, gas, chronic tiredness, inability to concentrate, and stomach pain, while outcomes from eating mindfully might include energy, wakefulness, and power.

6 If overeating is an issue, keeping a food diary either via an app on your phone (if your phone isn't a form of distraction) or in a notebook can help hold you accountable and aware of what you're consuming throughout the day.

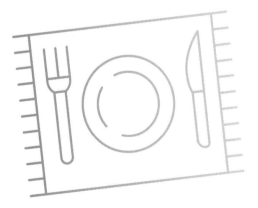

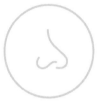

Smell

If only there could be an invention that bottled up a memory, like scent. And it never faded, and it never got stale. And then, when one wanted it, the bottle could be uncorked, and it would be like living the moment all over again.

DAPHNE DU MAURIER

(25)

The Calming Effect of Candles

Scented candles draw us in with their fragrance, but it turns out their allure and how they help calm the mind and body go beyond our sense of smell when they burn.

"It is scientifically proven that scented candles can play an essential role in the physiological effects of mood, stress, working capacity, and overall mental health," Chryssa Chalkia, an accredited clinical integrative psychotherapist (UKCP) and cognitive behavioral therapist based in London, shared in *Travel + Leisure* regarding the effect scented candles have on reducing anxiety.

Chalkia understands how important it is to make clients feel comfortable and relaxed when talking with a therapist, so she uses things like scented candles in the therapeutic room. "Scented candles have been used for centuries in all manner of rituals as they promote healing, enhance meditation and cleanse energies," she wrote in her article for Counselling Directory. "The gentle, mesmerizing quality of their light makes them a perfect aid for any relaxation routine."

Some people choose to use candles as a form of meditation or part of their yoga practice. According to *Yoga International* magazine, if you've ever been transfixed by a candle flame and felt your mind clear, you may have been tapping into a yogic focusing practice called *trataka*. Trataka, or *trataka sadhana*, has also been called candle gazing meditation because our eyes are concentrating on the flame, which in turn keeps our minds from wandering.

Amanda Glazebrook, founder of Pine & Burn Candle Co., isn't surprised more people are turning to candles to help get into a relaxation space. She started her business as a hobby and soon found friends and family wanting her candles. As a lover of romance novels, she created her line based on scents she felt best aligned with romance novel characters and the feeling of losing oneself in the characters and stories of this genre of books. Her website makes it very clear that Pine & Burn Candle Co.'s candles help keep your (book) crush burning, long after you've turned the last page. "Whether you lust after the gentle Horse Whisperer, who knows exactly when to go slow and when to go hard; the Dark Heart with a dangerous edge who can get you into (and out of) so much trouble; or the Pirate with an adventurous soul who searches the seas for booty (and love), we've got you covered," her About page, aptly titled "Romancing the Flame," notes.

Of course, how scents smell when her candles are lit

takes center stage. Glazebrook takes great care deciding which scents to use to create each candle, but there is another reason she loves candles in her spaces.

"There's sort of an inherent ritual to having a candle," Glazebrook told me. Unlike perfume, where you spray it and you have the scent on and with you, a candle requires some act of participation. If it's in a jar, you have to open the jar. You have to strike a match and hold the match to the wick. "There's this active participation and these moments of slowing down," she explained. "You have to pause and be with the candle when you're lighting it."

Since you're never supposed to leave a candle unattended, there's also a kind of passive tending that happens when you're burning a candle. "You check on it, you make sure everything's okay. You make sure it's burning cleanly. I like that aspect of it. It's an excuse to stop, slow down, focus on this one thing, even for ten to fifteen seconds."

Then there is the fire. Glazebrook feels there is something primal about the flame. As humans, we're drawn to the elements, whether it's earth, water, air, or fire. While we don't need candles to cast light or keep us warm, it's a nod to simpler times and before technology took over our lives.

The joy of having a candle is partly the scent, partly the act of lighting it, and partly having something that's warm and comforting to set the mood. The main reasons people are drawn to candles are their scents and the memories they evoke or the feeling people want to have in their space at that time. Glazebrook has a customer whose family is from India, and she bought one of her sandalwood fragrant candles because they remind her of home. "Every time she opens it up, she says it smells like India," Glazebrook said.

Glazebrook admits scents are very personal to people, and part of her business practice is to only include scents she personally loves. One scent she doesn't love is patchouli, but her husband loves it, especially with cedar. He asked her to make him a candle with those scents, so she did and he now burns it in his office. While she originally hated the scent, she now closely associates it with her husband, and it's grown on her.

"The soothing effect that candles have is based on how the brain processes smells," Chalkia said. "The smell of scented candles stimulates our limbic system, the part of the brain that is home to our memory and emotions. Hormones like serotonin and dopamine can be produced to help regulate mood. Therefore, our emotional state is influenced by the relationship that exists between scents, memories, and emotions."

——————— TRY IT ———————

There is a reason candles play a prominent role in a hygge lifestyle, a central aspect of Danish culture that's all about slowing down and finding ways to feel happier during the cold and dark winter months in Nordic countries. Candles literally light up a room when natural sunlight is scarce. Here are three things to consider if you want to add more scented candles to your life.

1 When seeking out candles, consider their scents and what type of feeling you're seeking. Chalkia recommends the following scents:

LAVENDER instantly relaxes both mind and body.

CLARY SAGE lifts mood.

CINNAMON makes you feel refreshed.

ORANGE reduces stress.

LEMON improves mood.

APPLE controls anxiety.

PEPPERMINT wakes up your mind and enhances focus.

FRANKINCENSE helps battle anxiety and gives great stress relief.

SANDALWOOD relaxes and calms body and mind.

VANILLA increases happiness levels, uplifts your mood, and stimulates feelings of relaxation and joy.

2 Ask candlemakers if they can recommend something based on what scents you like. Glazebrook happily shares recommendations based on what she has available, and if she doesn't carry a scent in her line, she'll recommend other candle companies. You may be surprised what's recommended to you.

3 Try lighting candles during different times and under different circumstances. Add a candle to a night bath routine, light one as you cozy up with a blanket and a book. You could also light a candle as part of your meditation routine or bring a candle to the dinner table. There is no right or wrong way to enjoy a scented candle. Sometimes I'll light one up as I'm doing dishes because it's comforting and I love the smell. Light it up whenever you feel the urge. It's a lovely and easy way to engage your senses and make you feel calm without a lot of effort.

Fresh from the Oven

There is no mistaking the fresh, earthy aroma of bread baking. Inhaling the scent can make us feel comforted, safe, and loved, since we often associate the scent with memories of when we were younger, being cared for by a loving family member who made sure we were well-fed and happy.

Jennifer Billock, author of *Historic Chicago Bakeries*, recently began baking bread as a hobby and appreciates the nostalgia. "Who didn't have a sandwich when they were growing up?" she joked. "You know what bread smells like when it's that close to your face."

Billock loves sweets so she started making dessert breads, which she admits are more batter-based than dough-based. She began experimenting with a no-knead country loaf before her brother gifted her a sourdough starter. With that starter, she baked an herb sourdough. "It smelled amazing in the oven and it tasted really good. But that smell, man, it was just so good."

Ellen King understands the power of scent and the whole process of baking bread. King is a baker, co-owner of Hewn Bakery in Evanston, Illinois, and author of *Heritage Baking: Recipes for Rustic Breads and Pastries Baked with Artisanal Flour from Hewn Bakery*. She calls the entire process of creating a loaf of bread therapeutic and a form of contentment, something she does just for her even though she owns a bakery.

"From the silence of working alone to mixing the ingredients, shaping it and baking it, to eating it," King explained.

While many of us do think about the warm scent while a loaf is baking, all the senses are at play when we're preparing and baking bread.

Unlike cooking a dish, which doesn't always require precision or following steps in a certain way, baking bread requires focus and following directions more closely in order to achieve a delicious final product. This feeling of being focused and your hands busy, actively doing something, helps us be present. There is literally no other way to bake bread. It demands your undivided attention.

"You're either mixing the bread, or you're shaping it, or you're baking it, and it's the touch, it's the smell, all your senses are captured by it," King added.

King loves watching something transform from simple raw materials to something delicious. We're taking flour and water and transforming it into an amazing baked loaf of bread that we can share.

"You just get lost in the process," she said. There are very few opportunities when we can get into the flow of something and we allow it to take over our time.

Baking bread forces you to slow down.

"You're on a bread's timeline," King said. "You can't speed it up. Even if you want to try and cut corners, you can't. You're working on the timeline of the bread and the yeast and the weather. You have to pay attention to what the weather is, if it's really cold in your kitchen. You want it to be the right temperature. All of it."

When you're baking bread, you're also committed to that project for a few hours. Depending on the type of bread you're making, you may have to return to it every half hour to turn the dough, shape it, or let it rest.

In an effort to harness the therapeutic benefits of baking bread, Bethlem Royal Hospital, a psychiatric hospital in Kent just outside London, created Bethlem Baking Buddies, a series of baking sessions for residents as a way to use bread baking as therapy. A report from the study found 100 percent of the residents felt happier and more creative, 80 percent were more relaxed, and 67 percent admitted feeling less anxious as a result of baking bread as an activity. Among the feedback one participant shared in the report: "Learning and making at the baking session helped me by lowering my stress and negative thoughts."

Baking bread is something we can do for ourselves or to share with others. It stimulates all five of our senses, and the act of sharing can help connect us. While there are a few things to learn before we can bake a perfect loaf of bread, once we figure out the details, we can give our minds a break from the noise and simply enjoy the process of watching the transformation of unbaked dough into a warm loaf.

─────────────── TRY IT ───────────────

1. Billock recommends starting with a no-knead country loaf recipe since you can use a mixer instead of having to knead it by hand. If you're just starting out, this might be a good way to get an idea of how baking bread works.

2. King understands the appeal of starting with a no-knead recipe, but she loves to get her hands into her dough. Once you get the hang of a no-knead loaf, take it to the next level by choosing a type of bread to bake. Spend some time reading through the recipe in advance, and consider the flavors and scents you might enjoy as the loaf is baking.

3. Baking bread doesn't require a lot of ingredients or equipment, but it does help to have a few things handy. King recommends a scale and a bench scraper and, while it's not necessary, a basket to put your bread in. You'll also want something sharp like a paring knife or kitchen scissors to score the bread to really get it to open up nicely when it's baking.

4. Like other things we try in life, don't give up after the first attempt. Billock almost guarantees your first attempt will be barely edible since it'll be pretty dense. "Don't put a lot of pressure on yourself," she advised. After you have baked your first bread and understand how it's done, try it again and see how much you've improved.

5. Once you get the hang of it, keep experimenting with different recipes and different artisanal flours. You'll soon find your flow and look forward to baking bread not only for the aroma as you're prepping the ingredients or while it's baking but also because you can share your loaf with others if you wish.

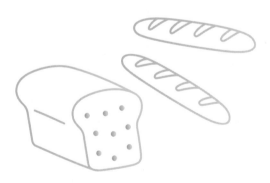

(27)

The Nostalgic Power of Perfume

It's not uncommon to be walking down a sidewalk or in a grocery store, get a whiff of someone's perfume or cologne, and the scent conjures up memories and certain feelings, even if those memories are from decades ago.

One of the reasons, said Sarah Horowitz-Thran, owner and chief perfumer of Sarah Horowitz Parfums, is our sense of smell is the strongest memory and emotional recall and is the only physical sense that bypasses the neocortex (thinking brain) and goes directly to the limbic system (primal brain).

"Because of this, smell is the only physical sense that bypasses thought and goes directly to feelings," Horowitz-Thran told me. "Scent can bring you powerfully into the moment without thought—and doing thus by using a fragrance that has a particular calming effect on you specifically, like your favorite scent or your mothers' perfume, can not only calm your mind but bring you into the present moment."

Sarah McCartney, London-based indie perfumer at 4160Tuesdays and coauthor of *The Perfume Companion*, takes the concept one step further and notes that our brains are constantly on the alert for something we can eat, someone who smells really good, and anything that could harm us. "We are reassured by aromas which remind us of safe places," McCartney added.

Unlike essential oils or candles that we use in our spaces, perfumes are even more personal because we wear them, we identify with them, and others smell them on us.

Perfumes also calm us and help keep us feeling safe and comforted.

Even when we're not conscious of it, McCartney said we use a lot of brain space exploring the aromas of somewhere new. "If you have favorite perfumes which always give you a good feeling, then you can wear them in an unfamiliar place to bring an atmosphere of safety with you," McCartney said. "If you are staying overnight in an unfamiliar place, no matter how restful and comforting it seems, your brain will be processing the new smells. Getting a good night's sleep the first time you stay there is almost impossible. It's as if your nose refuses to switch off. Bringing a favorite perfume and spraying the pillow will help to convince your brain that all these new olfactory experiences are nothing to be worried about."

Whenever she feels stressed or anxious and wants to feel calmer, Horowitz-Thran turns to her signature scent, one she has loved since she was eighteen. When she smells it, it reminds her of who she is and what she loves.

She also loves vanilla and sandalwood for calming and centering, with a hint of rose absolute, which is known for encouraging love of all kinds, including self-love.

Before McCartney started making her own fragrances, her pillow spray favorite was Shalimar by Guerlain. "It's a vanilla scent, so it brings the familiar comfort with it," McCartney said. "I also love Diorella by Dior, my first love, the scent I bought with my own pocket money when I was sixteen. It is so beautiful, it just makes me happy. It's like sitting down in my favorite chair."

Now that she has a collection of her own, McCartney uses one called Blue Screen Blue Horizon to calm down at night. "I made it as an antidote to spending too much time looking at electronic screens and not enough at the space where the sea meets the sky," she said. "For getting through the day, I use Meet Me On The Corner, a citrus chypre with a lot of fluffy musks and a nod to the unisex scents of my younger years. For exploring a new place when I can feel a slight rumble of uncertainty, I go with a floral amber fragrance named Truth Beauty Freedom Love because it helps me to remember the important things in life."

What some people don't realize about perfume and its power is that we tend to think we smell with our noses, while it's actually our brains that are doing the work when we respond to an aroma.

"The nose does all the collecting, but it's the brain which makes people feel differently, depending on what they are smelling," McCartney said. This is why when you're heading somewhere or doing something you want to distinctly remember and create a new memory, you want to choose your perfume wisely. That scent, McCartney said, will bring you back to that experience. It's also why we're drawn to different scents and feel happy around them, even if the scents aren't what you'd typically associate with "happy" or calming aromas.

"People are very much influenced by their own scent history," McCartney added. "When we smell perfumes, our minds search to recognize familiar aromas which please us. People can be drawn to completely different scents."

She shared the story of a woman she met who had spent a long time as a girl recuperating from a terrible accident at her grandparents' farm. For that reason, she adores "barnyard" or animalic scents that many people would find shocking. But for this woman, the familiar scent was comforting.

We're also drawn to familiar scents because they help calm our minds and bodies. And while most of us might know the scent of lavender as calming, one research study published in *Physiology and Behavior* notes the odor of oranges can also reduce anxiety and increase positive mood and calmness in women. Horowitz-Thran isn't surprised by the study's findings. "It has been known in aromatherapy that citrus notes, and orange in particular, can have a mood lifting effect," she said, noting that it's a natural antidepressant and stimulant. "I have found in my practice that lavender can be polarizing, as it is quite herbaceous, whereas orange is a bright, generally pleasing scent—clients smile automatically when they smell it."

"Orange and lavender are both balancing materials in that if you're too whizzy, they will calm you down, and if you're low, they will bring you up to a level state," McCartney said. "I have a mood fragrance, with several different orange essential oils, plus vanilla and cocoa absolutes, which I made to bring a feeling of calm to the evening."

―――――――――――― TRY IT ――――――――――――

1 Choosing a scent is very personal, but like choosing a wine you enjoy drinking, it doesn't have to be expensive, and you don't have to choose something trendy. Instead, allow yourself to enjoy the process and try different scents in different situations to see what you're drawn to.

2 In the book McCartney cowrote, *The Perfume Companion: The Definitive Guide to Choosing Your Next Scent*, she and her coauthor recommend you test a perfume before you commit, whether in a shop or via a sample. "Leave the atmosphere of the fragrance department and take it for a walk in the fresh air," they wrote. "First impressions change and generally you'll need at least twenty minutes with a new fragrance before you'll know whether you want to spend a couple of months with it."

3 Horowitz-Thran encourages those who want to use perfume as a way to calm their mind and body to be intentional about the experience. "I encourage an intentional process of stopping, closing your eyes, taking a few deep breaths, and inhaling the scent while you repeat a mantra that states your intention, which can be focused on relaxation, calming, soothing, or any other focus you set your mind to," she advised.

(28)

The Essentialness of Essential Oils

As the bath fills with water, it's the scent of lavender that calms me. When I need to rev up for a project, I take a whiff of peppermint or jasmine.

The nose-brain connection is so strong that it takes only a few sniffs of a scent to ease your mind, calm your body, help you focus, and put you in a good mood. Essential oils can be a helpful way to release tension and combat the effects of stress.

Essential oils have been in use for more than two thousand years. The trace of scent dates back to ancient Egypt, India, Persia, Mesopotamia, and China where essential oils were used to prevent illnesses or treat diseases and during religious ceremonies or rituals. They can be used in many ways including aromatherapy, massage oil, bath oils, and perfumes.

Aromatherapy is the practice of using essential oils for

therapeutic benefit. While essential oils have been used for centuries, it is René-Maurice Gattefossé, a French chemist and perfumer, who is credited with discovering the benefits of essential oils in 1910 when a laboratory accident burned his hands and he turned to lavender oil to treat it. He published the first book on the subject in 1928 and created the name we're familiar with today: *Aromatherapie.*

Today, there is mounting evidence, both anecdotally and scientifically, of how aromatherapy can play a role in supporting our mental health needs.

Essential oils are basically plant extracts made by steaming or pressing various parts of a plant (flowers, bark, leaves, or fruit) to capture the compounds that produce fragrance. Research suggests that when we inhale an aromatic particle, it triggers an immediate response in the brain that can influence our behavior and overall state of mind.

How and why does aromatherapy work? "When inhaled, the scent molecules in essential oils travel from the olfactory nerves directly to the brain and especially impact the amygdala, the emotional center of the brain," according to Johns Hopkins Health. "Essential oils can also be absorbed by the skin. A massage therapist might add a drop or two of wintergreen to oil to help relax tight muscles during a rubdown. A skincare company may add lavender to bath salts to create a soothing soak."

Aromatherapy can be an effective therapeutic option for the relief of depressive symptoms. One study measured the vital signs and levels of pain, anxiety, depression, and sense of well-being of seventeen cancer hospice patients and their responses to humidified essential lavender oil aromatherapy. The results reflected a small yet positive change in blood pressure and pulse, pain, anxiety, depression, and sense of well-being after both the humidified water treatment and the lavender treatment.

"The ability of essential oils to trigger different neural pathways without having the side effects of synthetic drugs makes them potential alternatives for treatment of mental illnesses including depression, anxiety, and dementia," wrote Lorena R. Lizarraga-Valderrama in her research published in *Phytotherapy Research.* "However, due to their synergetic effects and complex receptor-EO compound interaction, greater research must be done, especially in clinical research to promote the development and acceptance of EO-based drugs."

How aromatherapy is used can make a difference in how it's received. Another study, for example, noted aromatherapy massage had more beneficial effects than inhalation aromatherapy.

TRY IT

1. Start small. Pick three essential oils you are interested in based on the needs of you and your family, and learn more about them, suggest experts at University of Minnesota. Here are some suggestions to get you started:

   * Lavender is the powerhouse of essential oils. Research published in the journal *Frontiers in Behavioral Neuroscience* suggests that one fragrant compound present in lavender can lessen anxiety by stimulating the nose to pass signals to the brain.

✳ Some citrus scents, like lemon, and scents from herbs such as rosemary have been found to have a calming effect.

✳ Peppermint, jasmine, and sandalwood can be deeply relaxing.

2 Learn as much as you can about essential oils and how to best use them. The biggest misconception Maureen Anderson, DNP, RN, and Megan E. Voss, DNP, RN, licensed nurses with advanced training in aromatherapy at the University of Minnesota, see with aromatherapy is that consumers want to believe that a natural plant-derived substance is 100 percent safe. "In reality, these products are extremely potent," they said. "As much as they have the potential to provide therapeutic benefit, they also have potential to cause harm. Essential oils really can act like a medication in the body. They can cause allergic reactions and damage organs. They can even cause dangerous interactions with prescriptions or over-the-counter medications if used incorrectly." One example the Food and Drug Administration (FDA) offers is that cumin oil is safe in food but can cause the skin to blister. Certain citrus oils used safely in food can also be harmful in cosmetics, particularly when applied to skin exposed to the sun.

3 Make sure you're getting your information from a reputable source. The FDA classifies essential oils as food supplements, not drugs, which means producers of essential oils are not allowed to market the compounds as medicine. Companies that sell essential oils must clearly state the

product is "not intended to diagnose, treat, cure or prevent any disease." While the FDA prohibits companies that sell essential oils from providing clinical education or advice, according to the Dietary Supplemental Health and Education Act of 1994, this classification also means it is not allowed to regulate the sale or use of essential oils unless it can prove a particular product poses a serious threat.

4 Remember, less is more. Start with very small amounts of essential oils, Anderson and Voss recommend. "It is easy to add more, but it can be difficult to clear the air or clean the skin quickly if you use too much or too many essential oils and start to feel undesirable effects."

5 Finally, experiment with how you're planning to use essential oils. You can wear them as part of jewelry, add a few drops in a warm bath, or use them with a diffuser. You may find you love them in a bath but not so much in your living room. Also, keep in mind some essential oils can be toxic to pets, so it's a good idea to be mindful of which ones you use and where so as not to harm others at home who may be more sensitive to scents.

(29)

Nature Therapy

Being in nature may not seem remarkable, but a subtle shift happens when you step into a space where you're surrounded by nature's unfiltered beauty. For one thing, you may be alone and not see anyone else. There is something both uniquely comforting and terrifying about the idea of being alone. Many of us crave this alone time, not being tethered to our computer screens or electronic devices or within earshot of kids demanding our attention or spouses asking about dinner or whether we paid the bill or made a doctor appointment or whatever other thing we needed to do, forgot to do, didn't have time to do—you get the picture.

When we finally get the opportunity to *be alone*, some of us might get anxious. What if someone *was* trying to reach out because there was an emergency? Or what if something happened to *us*, like we trip over a branch and sprain our ankle and can't walk?

What if we could set aside those worries and for a moment just appreciate our surroundings? Realize that nature is awesome and expansive, and the trees are strong and grounded, and take a moment to permit ourselves to feel safe under their canopies. To feel nature's warm embrace. To be in awe of being where you are, soaking it all in, and noticing that everything is connected. We need the sun, the trees, the birds, and more. We rely on each other. We need trees in order to breathe. We need the sun so the trees can grow. Take a moment to reflect on the importance of nature to our ecosystem and our lives.

"Nature therapy means immersing yourself in the natural world by wandering while using all of your senses to connect with the natural elements around you," Brenda Spitzer, a certified forest therapy guide, explained.

Spitzer first learned of the real benefits of nature therapy more than a dozen years ago when she served as a trail patrol volunteer at the Morton Arboretum in Lisle, Illinois. "Being a trail patrol volunteer gave me a good and valid opportunity to slow down and be out in nature for two hours at a time," she told me. "During my shifts, I noticed that walking on the trails through forests and prairies helped me feel calmer and more centered."

She would go on to become certified to lead forest therapy walks, something she continues to do today. Through leading the walks, she's seen firsthand the powerful mental and physical health effects it can have on participants.

"When out in nature, our mental health is enhanced when we are pulled into the present moment," she said. "We are pulled into the present by breathing in the fresh air, using our senses to notice natural elements like fragrances, natural colors, textures, lines, and shapes, and watching movement in the environment. Being present in the moment makes us feel calm and connected to the world around us. Our physical health is enhanced by the simple act of moving through the environment."

Hundreds of scientific studies show interaction with nature is associated with increased happiness, social engagement, and manageability of life's tasks and decreased mental distress. Some researchers found that interacting with nature enhances cognitive functioning, while other researchers noted time in nature specifically increases working-memory span and improves mood.

And then there are the smells of nature that help ground us too! Smells experienced in nature can make us feel relaxed, joyful, and healthy, according to research. The study, published by *Ambio*, examined the role of smell in influencing well-being through nature and found that smells affected multiple types of human well-being, with physical well-being noted more frequently, particularly in relation to relaxation, comfort, and rejuvenation. That's not to say the absence of heavy scents is a negative thing. According to the study, the absence of pollution or unwanted smells in nature, especially in city landscapes or urban areas, can enable relaxation as well.

We don't need to spend hours in nature to reap the emotional and mental health benefits. Some studies suggest even short periods of time in nature can reduce symptoms of depression. Dutch researchers found that living close to parks, or at least near lots of trees, can have far-reaching mental health benefits for people. Conversely, living in places without parks or trees, especially if you are young or poor, can have major negative impacts.

Why Time in Nature Works

Nature takes us out of our heads, if you will, and reminds us that life is happening all around us all the time. We're not the center of the universe. We don't have to put all this pressure on ourselves to be the best, the fastest, the strongest, the smartest, the whatever it is you feel you need to be.

"When we are outdoors, immersed in nature, we have the opportunity to let go of our agendas and schedules and just use our senses to be present in the moment," Spitzer said. "For centuries, we humans spent most of our time outside, connected to nature. With the coming of the Industrial Revolution, technology, and factory production, most of us were pulled indoors for much of the day and lost much of our nature connection. Forest therapy walks give participants the opportunity and permission to let go of those to-do lists for a couple of hours and just be present together in the moment."

There is also tremendous comfort in the predictability nature affords us. No matter where we live, we usually experience some type of change in seasons or cycles. Many plants and some animals go dormant or retire to warmer climates in the winter, then spring emerges with hopeful new growth and a sense of renewal, followed by the heat of summer, only to wrap it all up with the slow pace of fall.

M. Amos Clifford, founder of the Association of Nature and Forest Therapy Guides and Programs and author of *Your Guide to Forest Bathing*, recognizes people have a hard time separating themselves from the device in their pockets. Instead of viewing your smartphone as an inherent evil, he recommends skillfully working it into a practice. "For example, if you're doing this slow walk around your garden or around the block, there may be a particular plant or scene. And you might decide, I'm going to photograph that [plant or scene] from standing at this spot every day for a year." When you stop to take a photo, take a moment to breathe in your surroundings, and take note of how everything around you smells.

At the end of the year, you'll have a year of photographs that you can enjoy viewing throughout the year but, more importantly, you'll connect with a sense of place in a way that is very powerful, according to Clifford. If you can leave your phone home or turn it off and enjoy your walk through nature, that'd be ideal. But don't let that be a deal breaker for time outdoors. "Instead, figure out how to use it in a disciplined way and where much of the time it's not present," Clifford recommended.

Spitzer agrees that leaving devices locked in cars if possible is preferable, but she also understands that may be too hard for some people. "If they need a device with them, as in the case of family that may need to reach them, I encourage them to silence their devices."

Richard Louv, author of *Last Child in the Woods: Saving Our Children from Nature-Deficit Disorder*, introduced the term *nature-deficit disorder* as a way to describe the growing gap between children and nature. "After the book's publication, I heard many adults speak with heartfelt emotion, even anger, about this separation, but also about their own sense of loss," he wrote in his follow-up book: *The Nature Principle: Reconnecting with Life in a Virtual Age.* Louv is also the cofounder and chairman emeritus of the Children & Nature Network and author of other nature-based books.

Louv makes a case for increasing our vitamin N (N for nature) in one of his books, adding that the mind/body/ nature connection will enhance physical and mental health. He argues the more high-tech our lives become, the more nature we need to achieve natural balance.

More time among nature helps us feel more alive, and he feels many of us desire a fuller life of the senses. According to Louv, we have the power to reverse our nature deficiency and increase our vitamin N. Our reliance on technology is a major culprit, and we need to disconnect to feel the power of our senses.

"Today, people who work and learn in a dominating digital environment expend enormous energy blocking out many of the human senses—including ones we don't even know we have—in order to focus narrowly on the screen in front of the eyes," Louv told me.

Ultimately, Louv said, this is about our ability to be fully alive. "As we focus for hours on our screens, we and our children spend much of our time and expend much of our energy trying to *block out* most of those senses so that we can concentrate on the screens a few inches from our eyes. To me, that's the very definition of being less alive. What parent wants their child to be less alive? What adult wants to be less alive? Some do, but most of us want something better.

"What do we miss seeing, hearing, and knowing because we allow the tangle of technology's wire to tighten around us each day?" Louv asked.

Like Clifford, Louv is not advocating ditching technology. He appreciates the benefits it provides, "but electronic immersion, without a force to balance it, creates the hole in the boat—draining our ability to pay attention, to think clearly, to be productive and creative."

So how does time in nature help us with this balance? Louv cited a study that suggests exposure to the living world can enhance intelligence for some people. "This probably happens in at least two ways: first, our senses and sensibilities are improved through our direct interaction with nature (and practical knowledge of natural systems is still applicable in our everyday lives); second, amore natural environment seems to stimulate our ability to pay attention, think clearly, and be more creative, even in our dense urban neighborhoods."

The best part of nature therapy is you don't need to drive an hour away to find an expansive forest to reap the benefits of forest therapy. Any green space where things are growing will work.

Clifford advocates for any time spent outdoors but encourages people to try a guided walk if provided the opportunity. He likens the experience to a yoga practice. While we can practice yoga at home, it's a different experience if you have a yoga instructor who can guide you, slow you down, and introduce you to the methods that really lead to the kinds of benefits that people report.

When I took a guided nature therapy walk with Spitzer, I was surprised at how often she had us stop and take in deep breaths. Most of us focus on what we're seeing around us, but we forget to inhale deeply and take in the scents. I've since taken the tips I learned from that guided walk and apply them daily. The benefits of taking a guided walk can't be underestimated—they are physical, mental, and often both. They include achieving a sense of calm, getting better clarity to think more creatively, or experiencing less depression or lower blood pressure. More importantly, though, Clifford said people who've participated in guided walks tell him they feel more connected to themselves, to the world, and to others.

"One of the principles we teach is that this is a practice," added Clifford. "It's much more about getting *here* than it is about getting *there*. And one thing that always enters us here, to this place, in this moment, is paying attention to our senses."

For those who are ready to try forest bathing, Clifford's book on the subject, *Your Guide to Forest Bathing*, can serve as a starting point. The Association of Nature and Forest Therapy Guides and Programs website features a map to help find the closest guided walk to you.

—————————— TRY IT ——————————

Whether you book time for a guided walk with a forest therapy guide or are ready to venture outside on your own, it won't be time wasted. Here are four ways to try it.

1   As if you were taking a walk around your block, start by dressing for the weather and wearing proper shoes. Before

you embark on your walk, make a concerted effort to unplug. Either don't take your phone with you if you think you'll be tempted to check it, or turn it off or silence it so the incessant dings of notifications don't distract you.

2. As you begin your walk, slow your pace. Stop, close your eyes, and inhale deeply. This isn't a marathon; it's a walk. Take your time, and allow yourself to engage all your senses, including your sense of smell.

3. As you continue your journey, slow your walk, and look at the trees more closely. If the trees are in bloom, look at the leaves and their veining. Touch the bark, and let your hands wash over the texture of the trunk. Breathe in the air, and see if you can smell the earth, the tree, the plants surrounding it. Can you hear the birds chirping? The rustling of squirrels as they run around and jump from tree branch to tree branch? Can you see the sun's rays peeking through the tree canopy or between homes as you continue your walk?

4. As you walk, notice how your body is moving and feeling. Are your arms effortlessly swinging by your sides, calmly? Are you noticing your muscles becoming less tense? Your heart rate less hurried?

5. Remember, it's not how long you spend in nature or how far you've walked that matters. Enjoy those deep breaths. Turn off your phone, get outside, and allow yourself the time to discover the healing power of nature to regenerate and restore.

30

Meandering

Ever had a moment where things just seem too much and you decide you need a breath of fresh air, so you head outdoors for a walk? Since we took those first few steps as babies, travel through walking offers us a way to experience the world at a slower pace, allowing us to take in everything around us.

Walking is also a great way to work through things with the benefit of movement. Being physically away from a computer screen or whatever issue you're needing to deal with and pounding the pavement with your feet opens the door to a level of clarity that doesn't always present itself in a different environment. For some, it can help ward off depression.

Joyce Shulman feels so strongly about the positive benefits of walking on the body and mind that she and her husband, Eric Cohen, started an entire business around the activity.

Shulman is cofounder, CEO, and self-described pack leader of 99 Walks, a wellness and walking lifestyle brand, community, and app on a mission to get a million women walking, and author of *Walk Your Way to Better: 99 Walks That Will Change Your Life.*

"The incredible thing about walking—an intentional walking practice—is that it is very powerful and impactful for your mind, your mood, and your body," Shulman told me. "It actually benefits all three of those systems in very meaningful ways. And in that way, I think it is just the perfect gateway to feeling better."

Part of why walking impacts our mental well-being is our brains process things differently while we're walking, enabling us to recognize what is truly holding us back and the changes we need to make, according to Shulman.

The positive benefits of walking for our bodies and minds are well documented. Research has shown that walking promotes the release of brain chemicals called endorphins that stimulate relaxation and improve our mood, according to the North Dakota State University Extension Service. What makes walking even more attractive as an activity is unlike intense physical exercise like running, which also releases endorphins and benefits your mind and body, you don't need to walk at a fast pace to enjoy those stress-relieving benefits. Even a short bout of walking lasting just ten minutes can improve mood in young adults when compared to no activity at all, according to one study.

Walking also activates another sense: our sense of smell. There is a good reason why we head outdoors for a walk, even if it's around the block, when we want to clear our heads. We can't help but take in the earthy aroma surrounding us no matter the season.

In her book *52 Ways to Walk*, Annabel Streets has an entire week (actually, several) dedicated to walking with the sense of smell in mind. In her week on taking a city smell walk (week 11), she recommends using our ears and eyes to seek out odor opportunities, from bakeries to florists and hedgerows to hospitals. And since the way a city smells changes by the season, she encourages us to try the same smell walk in the spring and then autumn, in heat and during rain, at dawn and at night.

Not every walk needs to be the same, and changing it up allows us to engage our senses. Some days, you may want to walk in the morning so you start it off on the right foot (pun intended). Other days, you may want to take a walk with a friend and use it as a way to catch up. There is no right or wrong way to go out for a walk to help calm your body and mind. It's all good. But allow yourself the time and space to meander and not be rushed to "get your steps in" for the day.

Shulman puts into practice four different styles of walks, depending on what she needs at any given time or day.

Shulman's Four Walks

1. Her first walk is walking with a friend, whether it's in person or on the phone. She feels so strongly about the connection that is formed when walking together that she dedicated a TED Talk around the theme.

2. The second is walking and losing herself in an audio-book or music she loves or really just getting lost in something when she needs that sense of escape.

3. Her third type of walk is when she wants time to focus on a particular challenge she's trying to sort out. "Like a puzzle, I'm trying to figure out what problem I'm trying to solve or a personal thing I'm trying to sort through," she said.

4. Her last type of walk is when she just wants to be outdoors and in nature, in silence, letting her mind wander and go wherever it'll go.

These four types of walks, she said, comprise an intentional walking practice that she puts into place daily.

Walking to Ward Off Depression

Walking as a regular practice offers many mental and physical health benefits, and for some, it can ward off depression, according to one study. The study sought to better understand whether being physically active can improve emotional well-being or if we simply move less when we feel sad or depressed, according to the study author, Karmel Choi, a clinical and research fellow at the Harvard T.H. Chan School of Public Health.

People who moved more had a significantly lower risk for a major depressive disorder—but only when the exercise was measured objectively using a tracking device, not when people self-reported how much exercise they performed.

"We saw a 26% decrease in odds for becoming depressed for each major increase in objectively measured physical activity," Choi said. "This increase in physical activity is what you might see on your activity tracker if you replaced 15 minutes of sitting with 15 minutes of running, or one hour of sitting with one hour of moderate activity like brisk walking."

Walking outside is something I do on a daily basis, and there has to be a really good reason for me to miss going out at *least* once a day. Having a dog who loves her daily walks helps me get out there, but even without her, I'll take any opportunity to get outside and breathe in the earth's smells. It makes me feel alive in a way few things can. I especially love how it smells after a good rain or in the spring when plants are coming out of hibernation. But even during the really cold Chicago winters, I'll grab my heavy winter coat, wrap my face with a warm scarf, and head outdoors because smelling that cool, crisp air revitalizes me (and I'm not one who loves the cold). I've never once regretted going outside for a walk, no matter the weather.

—————————————— TRY IT ——————————————

1. Wear proper shoes and socks. You don't need to invest in specific walking shoes, but a good pair of lightweight shoes with support and socks will help you feel comfortable as you take strides.

2   Wear appropriate clothing and gear. While it's natural for your body to warm up as you walk, especially if your walk is brisk, you'll still want to wear suitable clothing depending on the weather. Also, don't forget a hat and sunscreen.

3   Find a path. If your intent is to develop a daily walking practice, find a path you enjoy near your home or work. You're going to be more likely to go out for a walk if the route is aesthetically appealing.

4   Once you figure out a daily path (or a path you enjoy regularly), allow yourself to meander and not be so focused on completing your walk. Tune in to the scents around you as you meander. What is your nose picking up?

5   Consider your technique. Hold your head high, look forward, keep your neck and shoulders relaxed, swing your arms slightly (or use walking poles to help with stability and to get a full body workout while walking), and make sure you roll your foot from heel to toe as you take your steps.

6   Engage all your senses. As you walk, take deep breaths, feel the air, and take in the scents around you. Take a moment to hear the birds chirping. If you're in an urban environment and the sound of cars gets too loud, try to focus your attention on either the closest sound or the one farthest away. Feel the ground below you as your foot makes impact with the ground. Look at the living creatures, flowers, and fauna

around you. If you choose to take a bottle of water on your walk, sneak in a sip, and let yourself enjoy the hydration.

7. If your walking practice involves listening to audio like music, a meditation guide, or podcast, have that ready to go before your walk begins so you're not fussing with it as you're trying to walk.

8. Finally, enjoy the experience. Don't treat your walk as part of a to-do list, or you'll grow to resent it and not get the calming benefits it can afford. Instead, look at it as a way to give yourself permission to have some time to yourself, engage your senses, and enjoy your surroundings.

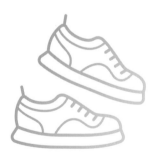

(31)

Smell the Roses

"Flowers are, unquestionably, the jewels of the green world," wrote Jan Johnsen, author of *Floratopia*. "Their sole task is to become pollinated and produce fruits and seeds, but it is the colorful and fragrant way they go about this task that captivates us."

Captivates us, indeed.

When I was planting flowers in my garden, I intentionally sought out fragrant plants near where I sit in the morning to journal because their scent is so potent at that time of day. I cannot wait to pour my coffee, grab my journal, and find my little space in my garden within inches of my jasmine vines that grow on one side of the trellis while the honeysuckle vines grow on the opposite side. Depending on the direction of the breeze, I'll get a whiff of one or the other's sweet scent. If I'm really lucky, I'll spot a hummingbird enjoying the sweet nectar each produces.

Researchers found that the smells from nature, including blooming flowers, affect multiple types of human well-being, with physical well-being noted most frequently, particularly in relation to relaxation, comfort, and rejuvenation.

Unlike other senses, smells are unique in the mechanism with which they affect cognitive processes and subsequently our emotions, memories, and perceptions of the world around us, the study reported.

Johnsen says aroma is food for the nose. "An average person draws 23,000 breaths in a day, and the scents contained in each breath convey information and provoke memories in a way nothing else can," she wrote in *Gardentopia*. "The effect of a scent is immediate because our sense of smell is connected directly to the limbic section (emotional responses) of the brain. It's no wonder that scent can control stress levels, heart rate and even blood pressure!"

This might explain why I love the scent of roses, either in the garden or in a bouquet on my kitchen counter. Roses, especially fragrant roses, are my mother's favorite plant. For years, my kids and I would buy her rose plants for her garden, and when I'd visit her and the weather was nice, she'd force me to take a walk through her garden (OK, *force* is a strong word, but she was always excited to have me see what was growing). She could recall which roses my kids or I bought for her and what year. She'd invite me to press my face against a newly bloomed rose and enjoy the sweet fragrance.

There is no way I can pass roses, whether in a grocery store or garden center, without stopping to quite literally smell the roses and think of her.

Flowers don't need to be outside to be enjoyed. We can also buy cut flowers for our homes or keep indoor fragrant houseplants to enjoy year-round.

Maria Failla, author of *Growing Joy: The Plant Lover's Guide to Cultivating Happiness (and Plants)* and host of the *Growing Joy* podcast, highly recommends adding fragrant plants to our indoor houseplant collection. And not just in the main rooms of your home but also within eyesight as soon as you wake up.

"Wake up, connect with plants in the morning, before you engage with your digital kind of universe," she said.

There are several houseplants that bloom and smell beautiful indoors, she told me. Rose-scented geraniums, *Maxillaria tenuifolia* (nicknamed "the coconut orchid" for its piña colada–scented blooms), lavender, and some hoyas are just a handful of examples.

One of my favorites are gardenias. When they're in bloom, my whole house smells like a botanic garden. During the winter, I love to grow amaryllis, and some have a wonderful scent. Paperwhites are another popular plant to grow indoors for their sweet-smelling flowers. And nothing screams spring is on its way to me more than showy and fragrant purple hyacinths.

If I don't have plants indoors for the summer (I usually take most of my houseplants outdoors when the weather is nice), I bring in cut flowers so I can still enjoy their beauty and fragrance while I'm working at my desk or having dinner with my family.

While Failla has been working with plants and flowers for several years, it wasn't until she began research for her book that she realized how little she was using her sense of smell when it came to her plant collection. She admits she was more focused on sight and how her plant collection looked.

I can relate. Foliage excites me too. I love my houseplants and seeing their greenery, especially during the dreary and cold months of winter. I don't always remember that some of my plants smell at all, let alone appreciate their fragrance, even if they're not always heady.

"There's so much that we've become disconnected from," Failla said in an understanding tone. "And I think in order to reconnect, you do have to foster those mindful moments of learning, reminding yourself to reconnect in that way."

"Flowers should play a bigger part in the modern world we live in because they brighten everyone's mood," Johnsen wrote in *Floratopia*.

I couldn't agree more.

—————————————— TRY IT ——————————————

1. If you want to introduce fragrant houseplants inside your home, consider scents you're drawn to and seek out flowers that have those types of scents. We shared a few in this activity, like geraniums, orchids, and hoyas, but there are so many others. "Remember, scent is personal, so choose what makes you happy, and check the care guides for your preferred plants before bringing them home," Failla added.

2. If you have outdoor space, Johnsen offers three ways to create a fragrant garden or add more scented plants to a garden. From her book, *Gardentopia*:

* Add fragrant plants near a door so you can enjoy a whiff as you enter or exit. I opted to place them where I journal every morning, but if near a door works better for you, this is a great suggestion.

* Grow fragrant plants near a sunny or south-facing wall. The reason for this location is heat encourages plants to release their scent. This might be why my vines are so fragrant in the morning—that and maybe the morning dew.

* Place your fragrant plants in an enclosed space such as a walled garden or small side yard so the scent can collect and stay in that area.

3. Make friends with your local florist! If you don't have time or the outdoor space to grow your own flowers and care for a plant indoors, use the opportunity to befriend your local florist and treat yourself to a bouquet every week or month or whenever you'd like. If you favor certain types of fragrances, your florist can also recommend flowers you might enjoy or let you know when they receive a special shipment.

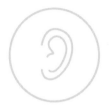

Hear

Silence is of different kinds, and
breathes different meanings.

VILLETTE, CHARLOTTE BRONTË

Mantra Meditation

There are one thousand ways to meditate. That is not a typo.

When most of us think of meditating, we think of someone sitting still, in the lotus position, and either focusing on their breathing or reciting a mantra.

I have a confession to make: I was among these people. I couldn't wrap my head around sitting still for any length of time and felt silly repeating a word or phrase over and over. It was through researching this book and reading studies that I decided to try it for a week—really try it—and see if I could silence the noise.

When you practice mantra meditation, you silently repeat a calming word, thought, or phrase to distract you from different things popping up in your headspace.

I was so unoriginal. I chose a simple mantra and a popular

one—a single syllable: the sound *om*. Some consider this syllable the original sound of the universe. I figured, why not? I enjoyed how it sounded when I exhaled it as well as when I released it silently. It reverberated in my head, and that hum felt so calming.

Meditation is a way to train our minds and helps us concentrate on the here and now—not the past, not the future. It gives us the tools to be less stressed and calmer when we feel life is out of our control. Regular practice is key because it prepares us for when we need to rely on this technique to get us through a hard time.

There is no shortage of studies that show meditation can be helpful when it comes to mental health problems, including mood and anxiety disorders.

Still, if you've resisted meditation in the past, as I did, there might be a good reason for this. Turns out the problem is most of us are just not comfortable in our own heads, according to a psychological investigation led by the University of Virginia. "In 11 studies, we found that participants typically did not enjoy spending 6 to 15 minutes in a room by themselves with nothing to do but think, that they enjoyed doing mundane external activities much more, and that many preferred to administer electric shocks to themselves instead of being left alone with their thoughts," according to research published in the journal *Science*. "Most people seem to prefer to be doing something rather than nothing, even if that something is negative."

"The mind is designed to engage with the world," Timothy Wilson, PhD, professor of psychology and public policy at University of Virginia and lead author of the study, said. "Even when we are by ourselves, our focus usually is on the outside world. And without training in meditation or thought-control techniques, which still are difficult, most people would prefer to engage in external activities."

Zen master and Buddhist monk Thich Nhat Hanh is considered the father of mindfulness, and Jon Kabat-Zinn is often credited with introducing mindfulness meditation to the masses.

Note that *mindfulness* and *meditation* are not interchangeable words.

Mindfulness, according to the Mayo Clinic, is a type of meditation in which you focus on being intensely aware of what you're sensing and feeling in the moment, without interpretation or judgment. Practicing mindfulness involves breathing methods, guided imagery, and other practices to relax the body and mind and help reduce stress.

Meditation doesn't always need to involve mindfulness. Meditation is an umbrella term for the many ways to achieve a relaxed state of being, according to the Mayo Clinic. Mantra meditation is just one way.

Meditation can be a powerful antidote to life's stressors, and practicing it daily means we can learn to focus our attention and choose how to respond to stressful situations when we need to. We're training our attention muscles to live a life with intention. Meditation allows us to engage and calm our minds and bodies, and its centering effects can help put us into a relaxed state, which will have positive ripple effects in our lives and those around us.

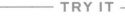
TRY IT

1 Figure out what kind of setting works best for you. If you feel

it's easier for you to sit on a cushion in a quiet room, make that your meditation space. The how isn't as important as setting aside time daily to practice.

2   Which leads to the second step: Set aside a dedicated time to meditate. Our minds wander easily, but if you set aside a dedicated time, you're more apt to keep your commitment to yourself. Some choose to start their day by meditating, while others choose to meditate and unwind at the end of the day.

3   Short on time? Even five to ten minutes helps. But eventually try to work your way up to meditating at least four days a week for twenty minutes.

4   Still feel like you can't meditate or you can't focus your mind? Try repeating a mantra, Mandisa Jones, LCSW, a licensed clinical social worker and founder of Ashe Counseling and Coaching, told me. "The mantra shouldn't have any meaning to it," Jones added. The mantra is meant to help you get into a flow or a trance-like state, and if other thoughts enter, which is totally normal, acknowledge them and return to the mantra. The more you practice, the easier it will be to get into that space next time you meditate.

5   Start slowly. If the idea of sitting still or meditating for twenty minutes doesn't sound possible, Jones recommends trying a class where someone guides you through a meditation. Or try it for just thirty seconds. Or a minute. "We can do anything for a minute," Jones said.

$$\text{33}$$

Feel the Beat

Think about any major event in your life, and you can probably connect it to a song. The first lullaby you sang to your child. The song you danced to on your first date. The song that comforted you when someone broke your heart. Your first concert with friends. The songs you chose to play during your wedding. The music played at a loved one's funeral.

It's been said that infants recognize the melody of a song long before they understand the words. Ever watch them as they try to mimic sounds and move to the beat of music as soon as they realize their bodies can move?

Listening to music has the ability to mend a broken heart, inspire us to move our bodies, encourage us to focus, motivate us to move faster, calm us down to go slower, connect us with a loved one, and help us wake up or go to sleep.

Research shows that listening to music can both relieve stress and elevate our mood. According to the NorthShore University HealthSystem, music can boost the brain's production of the hormone dopamine. This increased dopamine production helps relieve feelings of anxiety and depression. Music is processed directly by the amygdala, which is the part of the brain involved in mood and emotions.

According to researchers at Stanford University, "listening to music seems to be able to change brain functioning to the same extent as medication, in some circumstances." Music is one of the few things that is easily accessible to almost everyone, which makes it a practical stress reduction tool.

The researchers gathered with other scientists, ethnomusicologists, and musicians at Stanford's Center for Computer Research in Music and Acoustics in 2006 for a symposium to share ideas that push the boundaries of our understanding of the human musical experience. During the symposium, the scientists suggested that rhythmic music may change brain function and treat a range of neurological conditions, including attention deficit disorder (ADD) and depression.

Among the symposium participants was Dr. Harold Russell, a clinical psychologist and adjunct research professor in the Department of Gerontology and Health Promotion at the University of Texas Medical Branch at Galveston. Russell used rhythmic light and sound stimulation to treat ADD in elementary and middle school boys. "His studies found that rhythmic stimuli that sped up brain waves in subjects increased concentration in ways similar to ADD medications such as Ritalin and Adderall," wrote Emily Saarman for *Stanford Report*.

Jaime Alspach isn't surprised by the positive research around listening to music and the effects on our minds and bodies. As a music therapist of more than twenty years and cofounder of Music Therapy Enrichment Center, she's been using music as part of her therapy when working with clients on a daily basis.

"A lot of things are processed on only a single side of your brain, but everything we do is processed in individual places in the brain," Alspach told me. "When people are listening to music and their brain is being scanned, places on both sides of the brain light up. This allows firing between sides and can rebuild pathways that are broken after something like a stroke."

Formal music therapy can help some people alleviate pain, minimize stress, and ease symptoms of anxiety and depression. As a music therapist, Alspach works closely with patients using music as a tool to help them enrich their lives. Music therapists can help guide clients to make playlists, work with guided imagery, and match music to their current mood or use mood music to gradually get them to a calmer state.

When Alspach worked in a mental health and substance abuse hospital, often patients were anxious to be in a room with other people and to share anything about their lives. "In those settings, music was a thing for them to focus on that isn't invasive and is inclusive because it is just there," Alspach said. "For someone with anxiety, music meets them where they are at. It can pull you from that anxiety state and help you relax."

Just as much as music has the power to soothe and calm

us, hearing our favorite tunes or listening to upbeat music can improve our moods too. Research reveals a causal link between dopamine and the reward response in humans when listening to music. In fact, it doesn't take long for that happiness to kick in when listening to great tunes. Another study published in the *Journal of Positive Psychology* found people who intentionally listened to upbeat music improved their moods and happiness in just two weeks.

Others find plugging in their headsets to be an important part of their exercise routines that helps motivate them to get to the gym, or they use the repetitive beats of the songs on their playlists to help them power through a long run.

Making Music

While listening to music can be powerful, making it can work wonders too. Making music has been shown to help reduce stress, lower blood pressure, and decrease your heart rate.

Ava Petlin listens to punk music because she likes the distraction it affords her. Punk music is her go-to, and she can spend about four hours a day listening to what she calls pretty aggressive music. She's drawn to the lyrics and the melodies. And when Petlin is stressed or needs a break, she turns to her guitar and strums out some country music songs.

"It's a good distraction, especially when I'm stressed, to focus on the notes in the music," Petlin told me.

She spends about an hour a day playing her instruments and rotates them depending on her mood and the type of music she wants to play. She alternates between an acoustic guitar, an electric guitar, and a bass guitar.

"If I wanted to play some calmer, like finger-style music, I'd normally pick up an acoustic guitar," Petlin noted. "But if I wanted to get some anger out, I'd plug in my electric or bass and start playing that."

For Petlin, the physical work of her hands on an instrument and listening to the music she creates puts her in an almost meditative state. She appreciates the repetition required to learn something and then the satisfaction from being able to play it back.

Get More Music into Your Life

For those who want to incorporate more music into their lives, experts recommend we consider what types of music we like to listen to for the situation at hand. If you normally want to wind down after a long day of working and you find slow and calming mood music helpful, start by creating a playlist of that type of music. Or maybe something more upbeat is preferable so you can shake off the day and start transitioning to a more fun evening. Creating more than one playlist for different scenes in your life is advisable, so when you're in need of something based on your mood, you have something at the ready.

I'm the kind of person who needs really fast-paced music while I run or do any sort of cardio workout, and I'm not alone. An article published in *Scientific American* noted that for "some athletes and for many people who run, jog, cycle, lift weights and otherwise exercise, music is not superfluous—it is essential to peak performance and a satisfying workout." Not only does the music help get my heart rate up and in the mood to push myself harder, as the article pointed out as well, "music distracts people from pain and fatigue, elevates mood, increases endurance, reduces perceived effort and may even promote metabolic efficiency. When listening to music, people run farther, bike longer and swim faster than usual—often without realizing it." The article cited a 2012 review of the research by Costas Karageorghis of Brunel University in London, one of the world's leading experts on the psychology of exercise music, who wrote that one could think of music as "a type of legal performance-enhancing drug."

There is no doubt that music can provide us comfort, bring back memories, capture an important moment, and soothe us. Music tells stories. Whether through lyrics or simply the progression of chords in a song, we can almost always find songs that we relate to in some way.

Listening to songs that evoke emotions and that we can relate to can be a great way to work through our emotions, thoughts, and experiences.

--- TRY IT ---

1 Start pulling together a playlist. Don't overthink what you include. Consider the type of music you like, and start creating different playlists based on the mood you feel when you listen to that genre or type of music. Want something more soothing and relaxing? Find some artists or music that help you feel calm when you listen, the kind of music that will quiet your mind and relax the muscles in your body. Usually this is music with a slower tempo, but maybe it's something different for you. Looking for something to get your mood up

or motivate you to work out? Perhaps you want to find pieces with a faster tempo.

2. Not sure what you want? Take the time to listen to different types of music, and see how they make you feel. Petlin has advice for those who might have a bias toward a certain genre: "Be open to listening to different types of music, because you never know what you would like."

3. Start listening to music as part of a daily habit, perhaps while you're brushing your teeth or taking a shower. It could be as simple as playing some music in the background while washing dishes or enjoying a meal.

4. If you want to try your hand at playing music, know that you don't need to be musically inclined to enjoy the benefits. Choose an instrument you enjoy listening to, and get acquainted with it and the sounds you create using it. Realize some instruments take more time than others to learn or master. If you're looking for something more immediately gratifying, choose a harmonica or drums over a guitar. Or if you know how to read music and understand the layout of piano keys, take up piano. Make it a point to play your instrument regularly so you get the benefit of playing and listening to the sounds it produces while improving your skills as well.

5. Finally, don't forget live concerts! Grab some friends, and make plans to go hear some live music on your own.

(34)

White Noise

Valentina Valentini, whose mind tends to race at bed-time, began using white noise to help her fall asleep using a free app on her phone. The London-based writer told me she needs some sort of noise to help the actual noise in her brain quiet down.

"I have the type of brain that can think about twenty different things at one time," Valentini said. "And just because I put my head on my pillow, even if I've read a book for twenty minutes and sprayed sleep aromatherapy on my pillow and snuggled up to my fiancé, my mind doesn't turn off. In fact, once my body is quiet and in the bedroom, things can get even worse in my head. I'll start thinking about the past a lot or what stresses are coming tomorrow. So white noise gives me something external to concentrate on."

White noise consists of a mix of frequencies played together at the same intensity level. Some people consider the sound of an electric fan or any sort of static sound as white noise. There are white noise machines, also called sound machines, where you can adjust the type of white noise you want to hear, or you can pull up white noise on your phone or computer to play as background noise. The idea is the white noise drowns out nearby sounds or gives your brain something else to focus on, so it gives it a break from the other "noise" in your head.

Dr. Jennifer Mundt is a sleep psychologist who is board certified as a diplomate in behavioral sleep medicine. She is an assistant professor of neurology at the Northwestern University Feinberg School of Medicine and a member of the NU Center for Circadian and Sleep Medicine. She isn't surprised some people, like Valentini, turn to white noise to help them fall asleep as she often hears from her patients, especially those who suffer from insomnia or mention they can't shut off their brain at night, how mental white noise can help to calm their body and mind and drown out those racing thoughts.

Not all white noise devices produce static sounds. Some produce ambient and natural sounds like rain, ocean waves, or chirping birds. Valentini used to fall asleep listening to a bedtime nursery album when she was young, and she said she's always needed a bit of noise to help her fall asleep.

How the brain reacts to white noise compared to other sounds is similar, but according to Joanna Scanlon, MSc, a researcher at the Mathewson Attention, Perception, and Performance Lab at the University of Alberta, it treats speech or songs differently.

"One EEG study found that white noise induced brain activity with lower amplitude to that of pure tones, but also higher amplitude to that of clicking sounds," Scanlon told *Bustle* in an interview. According to Scanlon, the study implies that the brain thinks the white noise is less worthy of attention than pure tones but more relevant than random clicking. This is why white noise machines help lull your brain to sleep—white noise masks the random noise of the street outside or your radiator tapping to life but isn't annoying enough to register in your brain.

A few years ago, Valentini's fiancé bought her a white noise machine, which—she finds funny—is white. She noted it is a little more sophisticated than her iPhone and has quite a few different options for sounds, including sounds like ocean waves, rainstorms, and the like.

Since the noise is nothing but repetitive sounds, concentrating on those repetitive sounds is what helps to quiet her brain. The white noise machine's variety allows her to change the sounds so the noise doesn't become monotonous and boring.

"I do like to switch it out sometimes and listen to rain," she added. "Never ever the crickets. That's just crazy. But now I pretty regularly use the white noise every night. The only time I might not use it is when the dehumidifier is on."

Mundt finds that patients tend to fall into two camps when it comes to white noise, and a lot of it is based on personal preference and subjectivity. "People either need silence, or silence is uncomfortable and they need some kind of noise," Mundt said.

─────────────────── **TRY IT** ───────────────────

1 Before investing in a white noise machine, check out white noise sounds online or through an app. There are a number of different sounds and settings for different lengths of time, so you can experiment with various types of white noise, nature sounds, or even music. As Mundt noted, there is no right or wrong type of white noise. Each of us is different, and you may need to try several before you find one you prefer.

2 If you do decide to invest in a white noise machine, there are several on the market, and most cost less than $100. Some have a basic, utilitarian design while a few have a high-design minimalist look. Higher-end models might offer a wider selection of sounds and volume dials.

3 Sound machines don't usually take up a lot of space, but for those who need something smaller, there are portable options. Also, some double as alarm clocks.

4 Be sure to check out the timers for any devices you're considering. Some machines will turn off after a certain period of time while others play on a continuous loop.

5 If you're planning to use a white noise machine at night, consider starting it about thirty minutes before you go to bed so you can signal to your body and mind to "turn off" and get you ready for a good night's rest.

Breathe In, Breathe Out

We all breathe. We have to in order to stay alive. But what is it about breathing deeply, listening to our breath, and the practice of breathing exercises that helps our bodies and minds?

The answer dates back to prehistoric times. When our prehistoric ancestors faced danger, they'd either flee or fight. In modern times, when we get stressed, our bodies still release cortisol, and the result is an increase in heart rate and energy due to this fight-or-flight response. Once the threat of danger is over, our bodies can return to normal breathing.

Breathing allows us to let air flow to our lungs and brings oxygen to our bodies so they can work properly. When we're under stress, whether due to danger or just being mentally, physically, and emotionally overwhelmed, it's no surprise that our breathing changes. Not only can we feel it in our bodies—our chests might tighten as we hold our breath or take faster and shorter breaths—but we can also hear our breathing changing as it tends to become shallower. This causes carbon dioxide to build up in our bodies, which then induces distress on the nervous system.

When you breathe deeply, you're helping to lower your blood pressure because you're tricking your body into thinking you're safe, according to Mandisa Jones, LCSW, a licensed clinical social worker and founder of Ashe Counseling and Coaching. There are different types of breathing techniques for stress relief. Belly breathing, box breathing, alternate nostril breathing, and lion's breath are just a few.

One of the reasons Jones recommends meditation to her clients is because the practice often incorporates deep breathing. If you've already developed a practice of meditation, then you're going to trigger that automatic breathing response.

"You trained yourself to breathe, to slow down," Jones told me. "And so when you are confronted in situations, then the breathing will be automatic. You're giving yourself a choice to breathe."

Or if you're noticing anxiety is creeping up because you're recognizing the physical responses such as tightening of your chest, sweating, or difficulty breathing, you have to consciously remind yourself to breathe, according to Jones. Again, this is where your breathing and meditation practice comes in handy because you've been practicing this scenario.

"When you are finding yourself with those anxiety symptoms, then you need to remember to breathe," she said.

Deep breathing is a grounding technique. There are a

number of different methods you can try to find one that works for you. The box breathing technique, sometimes called square breathing, works by having you count to four for a total of four times (a square box has four sides, hence the name box or square breathing). Listen and focus on your breathing. Begin by counting to four as you inhale slowly, hold your breath for four, then four counts as you exhale. Repeat four times: four-four-four-four. Breathe. Listen to your heart beating. Listen to your breath inhaling and exhaling. Feel your chest fill with air as you inhale and your belly sink into your body as you exhale.

Another grounding technique that involves breathing is the hand-on-heart five-steps exercise, which involves all your senses, from hearing to sight. According to the University of Rochester Medical Center, this five-step exercise can be very helpful during periods of anxiety or panic by helping to ground you in the present when your mind is bouncing around between various anxious thoughts.

"Though anxiety is often linked to thoughts, it's also a physical sensation, like hunger," Melissa Nunes-Harwitt, LMSW, a mental health clinician at Behavioral Health Partners with the University of Rochester Medical Center, shared on a YouTube episode regarding the hand-on-heart technique. "You can't think your way out of being hungry. You have to do something about it with your body." Hand-on-heart is a physical way to slow your anxiety and racing mind, Nunes-Harwitt noted.

To practice the hand-on-heart breathing technique, begin by paying attention to your breathing. Take slow and deep breaths to help calm your body and mind. Once you connect to your breathing, follow these steps:

5. Acknowledge FIVE things you see around you. It doesn't matter what you notice—just glance around the room and take stock of what you see. It could be a piece of artwork, your desk, the paint color on the wall. Anything counts.

4. Acknowledge FOUR things you can touch around you. Again, it doesn't matter what you touch. Touch your shirt, the chair you're sitting on, a pen on your desk.

3. Acknowledge THREE things you hear. Focus on external sounds, not your internal voice. Can you hear cars outside? Birds chirping? The sound of a washing machine?

2. Acknowledge TWO things you can smell. By now, you're getting the point of this exercise. Inhale and identify what you can smell. If you're indoors, can you smell the scent of your dish soap or a pillow in your bedroom? Can you venture outdoors and smell nature?

1. Acknowledge ONE thing you can taste. Can you taste anything inside your mouth from earlier in the day, like the taste of coffee or what you had for lunch? Or can you chew on some gum?

A study referenced in an article published in *Greater Good Magazine* reveals that several brain regions linked to emotion, attention, and body awareness are activated when we pay attention to our breath.

Paced breathing methods, like the box breathing and hand-on-heart techniques discussed earlier, require us to inhale and exhale with intention and to a set rhythm.

"This study found that paced breathing also uses neural networks beyond the brain stem that are tied to emotion, attention, and body awareness," the article noted. "By tapping into these networks using the breath, we gain access to a powerful tool for regulating our responses to stress."

The great thing about deep breathing is it's always available to you, twenty-four seven. You can do it anywhere, and no one needs to be the wiser. Only you can hear yourself breathing, so you can even do it around others. You can do it as part of a meditation practice or yoga. You can do it on the subway, while sitting at your desk, or while at a dinner party with your uncle who is asking you *again* if you're dating anyone.

——————————— TRY IT ———————————

To appreciate the benefits of deep breathing, it's best to make it a habit before you find yourself needing it. As with any habit you're trying to make (or break), it's best to connect it with another activity so you're more likely to do it. If you regularly sit at a desk to start your workday, try starting a deep breathing exercise as soon as you sit down. Or if you have to pick up your kids from school every afternoon, drive to your destination ten minutes early so you can do some breathing exercises.

1 First, try different types of deep breathing exercises to see which ones you enjoy doing. There are several different ones, and we've only outlined a few here. Some involve lying down while others you can do while sitting. Take the time to listen to your body and see what it needs.

2 If you opt for one in a seated position, sit in a chair with your back straight.

3 Slowly breathe in, and feel your lungs filling from the bottom to the top. Take a moment to listen to your breath or heart beating.

4 When you're ready, allow yourself to exhale slowly. Listen to the sound of the breath leaving the body. Feel your diaphragm relax as you empty your lungs.

5 Repeat throughout the day and on a daily basis to really gain the benefits from this activity. Practicing daily will make it easier to activate the exercise if and when you find yourself in a situation where you need to slow your breathing.

(36)

Calls of Nature

There is ample evidence to suggest that time in nature can be very beneficial to our bodies and minds. Whether it's a simple walk around the block or through the forest, allowing yourself that time to soak in all nature has to offer is a tremendous gift to your senses and reduces stress-related hormone levels. Listening to birds chirping, watching them fly or rest on a tree branch, and inhaling the fragrant scent of earth or feeling the fresh breeze on our skin helps us get out of our thoughts and appreciate our environment.

Christine Esposito, director and lead curator of Third Coast Disrupted: Artists + Scientists on Climate, admits she's always been a nature type and appreciated birds—especially their singing—for many years. "It's a way to connect—with the present, nature, the seasons, a place, the world around us, others," she told me. "When you're observing a bird, or trying to, you are wholly in the moment."

Bird-watching, or birding, surged in popularity during the COVID-19 pandemic as birds were not on lockdown, according to a *New York Times* article. "According to the Cornell Lab of Ornithology, birders set a world record on May 9 [2020] for Global Big Day, an annual bird-spotting event. Participants using the lab's eBird platform reported more than two million observations—the most bird sightings documented in a single day—and recorded 6,479 species."

There are several reasons Esposito loves the activity of birding that go beyond simply watching them.

"Birding is a way to channel curiosity and even a sense of adventure; you never know what you'll see," Esposito added. "You know what you hope to see or what you have a good chance of seeing, based on what birds are in the area, but there are often surprises."

Birding makes Esposito feel connected, awed, thrilled, exhilarated. "The sense of connection comes from being in the moment, which you have to be if you're going to get your binoculars on a bird or discern its song," she explained. "It comes from witnessing the beauty and wonders with others. It comes from being in nature, whether that's on your street or in a preserve."

For those who suffer from anxiety or are unsure of what to do when they're outdoors, bird-watching gives them something to do, according to Christopher W. Leahy, author of *Birdpedia*.

"Once introduced to the possibility of looking for and

identifying different bird species, this problem is solved," Leahy noted in an article focused on the psychological benefits of bird-watching. "And once the avian objective is identified, the rest of nature tends to enter the picture."

In a *New York Times* article, Layla Adanero mentioned how bird-watching became a respite for her faster-paced lifestyle she had to leave behind when COVID-19 hit. Adanero described listening to the sounds the birds make, the chirps and coos in her backyard, as clues to understanding an entire ecosystem.

"It's quite meditative to watch another life form go about its day," Adanero said. "It's like another way of practicing mindfulness."

While bird-watching, Esposito takes the time to appreciate the feat that some birds achieve, especially during migration. She pauses to reflect that a bird—sometimes weighing only a few grams—on a journey of thousands of miles during migration is something truly remarkable. "Many of the warblers are just stunning in their spring breeding plumage, little jewels of brilliant colors," she remarked with a sense of awe. "It's a privilege to see them and witness their trek. There's the thrill of identifying a bird for the first time, piecing together the clues until you figure it out. There's the exhilaration of spotting a bird that's rare for the area."

While watching birds can make someone feel awe and wonder, findings published in *BioScience* in 2017 note that, particularly for people living in an urban setting, "more bird species in the environment and watching birds have been shown to be good for people's psychological well-being, whereas listening to bird song has been shown to contribute toward perceived attention restoration and stress recovery." As Marta Curti reminds us in her article on the therapeutic benefits of bird-watching for *BirdWatching* magazine, in times of stress or even grief, "ornitherapy" can provide comfort and healing in surprising ways.

"Birding, by its very nature, teaches us patience and gently coaxes us into calm," Curti wrote. "Loud noises and quick movements will frighten most birds away. Thus, observing birds in the wild begs for stillness and silence—skills that, once learned, can help us in other trying situations. Searching for birds also demands our full attention. A quick look at our phone or a thought that sidetracks us might mean a missed opportunity to spot a bird before it takes flight."

Esposito agrees. Engaging most of her senses is critical when it comes to birding. "You're listening a lot more than some may realize," she added. "Often you'll hear a bird before you see it." Some birders excel at identifying birds by their calls and songs. Esposito has a background in music, which helps her.

Still, she said, you don't need a background in music to get the benefit of birding. "Some people aren't as adept at birding by ear, but they're awesome birders," she explained.

According to Curti, once we notice a bird or a bird is in our sights, there are any number of things that might hold our attention. "For some, it might be the movements of the bird— the flitting of a sparrow or the regal soaring of a hawk—that holds them rapt," she wrote. "Others might prefer to focus on the colors—whether it's the bright red of a Northern Cardinal contrasting with the green bush in which it perches or the muted palette of a female Red-winged Blackbird. Others still might prefer to focus on the sounds, such as the watery notes of a Common Raven or the ruffling of a Turkey Vulture's feathers. It isn't what we choose to focus on that matters but rather the simple act of mindfulness."

Birding is accessible to anyone and doesn't cost much to enjoy, and birds are everywhere. As Curti reminds us in her article, whether you live in the mountains, by the sea, in the desert, or near the neon-lit streets of a major city, you can find birds nearby.

─────────────── TRY IT ───────────────

1. Take a walk alone, if you feel comfortable and safe doing so. Or find a spot indoors so you can see through a window. You can bird-watch anywhere, including you own backyard or simply walking around you neighborhood. "During migration, if you happen to live along a migratory flyway, the birds are definitely there," Esposito said. "We just need to notice them. Even local year-round birds are worthy of observation. Sometimes we take them for granted, but they're beautiful and interesting too."

2. Once you spot a bird, take a moment to actively focus on hearing or seeing it. Once it comes into your sight, pay attention to its feathers and wings, its behavior, its song, or its calls, and listen for a response from another bird. Whether you're seated indoors or walking outside, don't rush what's happening in front of you.

③ Let yourself take a deep breath and enjoy the birds and the birdsongs. Even if you can't see them easily, pause when you hear a bird, and before you know it, you'll start to recognize each one's unique sounds.

④ While birding can be done solo, there are organizations or groups that organize bird-watching activities or bird walks. Many are free to join or participate in, and if you don't own binoculars, some groups make them available. "The walks are a great way to get your feet wet and meet some folks," Esposito said. "Most birders are happy to share their love of birding with others." Additionally, according to Leahy, "birders are a community and while birding in solitude can be a great form of meditation, it can also be emotionally rewarding to share a (non-stressful) relationship with those who share your passion."

⑤ If you're using binoculars, first spot the bird with your naked eye. "Then leave your head where it is, and bring the binoculars up to your face," Esposito advised. It's important to remember that using binoculars to find a bird takes practice, but it comes more easily over time.

⑥ Finally, don't give up if you can't immediately see birds, especially ones you don't see regularly in your area. "Spring warblers are constantly moving, flitting about often high in the trees in search of food," Esposito said. "The best way to spot them is to keep an eye out for their movement, instead of for the birds themselves. Once you know a bird's general vicinity, you can zero in on its location and hopefully get your binoculars on it."

Bathing
in Sound

There are very few things we can do to help calm our minds and bodies where we do not have to do anything but receive the experience. A sound bath, also known as sound therapy, is one of those things.

"Sound healing or therapy is the use of sound frequencies to affect the brain and the autonomic nervous system—calming the fight-or-flight response and resulting in relaxation, healing, and individual enrichment," explained Joanne Dusatko, a sound healing and therapy practitioner and founder of Sound Healing Remedies.

Why is the term *sound bath* used? Because a person is simply letting the sounds wash over them and bathe them. Unlike other activities like journaling, practicing yoga, or even doing a puzzle, you don't have to do anything to enjoy sound healing or have any previous experience or knowledge. "They just lie there, relax and receive," Dusatko told me. "Plus, the sounds can be cleansing and renewing, like a nice water bath."

Sound therapy can be done using singing bowls, crystal bowls, gongs, or bells, among other instruments. Dusatko has been a musician for most of her life and began using percussion instruments and her guitar to aid her practice of prayer and meditation. After discovering their power in group prayer and meditative settings, she decided to advance her skills and move into using sound for healing and stress reduction. She completed a 186-hour sound healing and therapy certification course that covered the full range of how sound affects us physically, mentally, emotionally, and spiritually.

Eventually, she began doing personal one-on-one sound baths for people where she would use percussion, singing bowls, vocals, tuning forks, and her guitar.

"People experience peace and serenity and often do not want to leave," Dusatko said. She decided to take her practice further and began offering group sound baths. During the group sessions, she includes more instruments: bowls, gongs, a tongue drum, frame and buffalo drums, Native American flutes, a zither, chimes, and a variety of shakers, rain sticks, bells, and other percussion instruments.

Several scientific studies provide evidence that music reduces stress and can improve one's mental state, but few focus on the effects of singing bowls or gongs. Still, the few studies done do show promising results.

One observational study published in the *Journal of Evidence-Based Complementary Alternative Medicine* found significant beneficial effects of Tibetan singing bowl meditations on a number of markers related to well-being, including mood, anxiety, pain, and spiritual well-being.

According to the study, the "authors set out to examine the possibility that merely lying down and listening to the high-intensity, low-frequency combination of singing bowls, gongs, and bells in a sound meditation could induce a deep relaxation response and positively affect mood and sense of well-being." What they learned is that compared with premeditation, the sound meditation participants reported significantly less tension, anger, fatigue, and depressed mood following the session.

One reason Dusatko believes sound therapy is so effective is because our bodies are 70 percent water, and water is an excellent conductor of sound. Also, everything is in a state of vibration, including our bodies.

That vibrating feeling can be profoundly effective, especially if you're the person engaging with the instrument. While most of the time, people experience a sound bath through a guided meditation or as part of a yoga practice, you can also buy and use a singing bowl at home.

Barbara Senn is an artist and first learned about singing bowls when she worked at a fair-trade store in Milwaukee, Wisconsin. She would start one bowl, then another, and another, and when one would stop, she would start it again.

Senn is drawn to both the sound and the feeling in her body when she engages with the bowl. She talked almost poetically as she explained how she takes the rubber mallet to the metal singing bowl (she prefers the metal ones instead of the crystal bowls) and hits it to hear the sound. Large ones, she said, can reverberate for several minutes, and you can have a full-body experience.

"You're standing and you're feeling it all over you, through one arm, through your chest area and down to your other arm," she said of her experience hitting a larger bowl recently. "It was really impressive."

She's drawn to singing bowls because they help her feel like she's centering herself, especially when she's going through difficult times in her life. They help drown out the noise, especially when she's experiencing anxiety. And as an artist who likes working with her hands and touching things, she's finding that she also likes the physical intimacy she has with objects because they make her feel more connected.

There's a reason Senn feels like this when she plays a singing bowl. The frequencies work through a method of entrainment, Dusatko explained. "They can synchronize our brain wave state. The frequencies of the bowls and gongs change the brain wave state from our usual alert beta state of problem-solving to the relaxed state of alpha and even the more dreamlike state of theta, with the possibility of going even deeper into the delta range, which can be very healing. The vibrations and frequencies of bowls and gongs activate the parasympathetic nervous system of the body, which results in decreased muscle tension, blood pressure, heart rate, and breathing rate."

Also, the tones increase the release of melatonin, endorphin, and dopamine chemicals that help to focus the mind, foster stronger concentration, and balance moods while reducing fatigue. This is why many feel a mental freshness after their session is over. "Group sound baths using crystal and metal singing bowls and gongs have a similar result of brain wave entrainment," Dusatko noted. "The result is often a calmness instead of a racing mind, a release from anxiety and deep relaxation."

As more people are learning about the calming effects of sound healing, whether introduced to it in a guided yoga class or seeking it out by purchasing a sound bowl to try at home, Dusatko encourages first timers to try a group sound bath first.

There is power in a group of people experiencing the same thing together. "The sound quality of the live event will also be excellent, and people can feel the vibrations through the air and sometimes even through the floor, thus receiving the full benefit of the vibrations," she explained. "When hearing a sound bath online, the sound may come through a computer speaker or phone, and the full range of vibrations and frequencies will not be experienced."

Although Dusatko may say she's a "sound healer," she admits it may be more accurate to say she's a "sound facilitator." It is the person receiving the sounds and vibrations who is really doing their own work of restoration, healing, and positive movement. "I am only providing a vehicle with my sounds and intent," she said.

If you decide you want to buy a singing bowl and are not sure which one to buy, Senn recommends trying them out in person, if you can, because the one that works for you will become obvious. "It's like, how do you pick out a pet? When you know, you just know," Senn said.

TRY IT

1. Approach the sound bath experience with curiosity and an open mind. Our thoughts are powerful and can affect the outcome of an experience. If you go into it full of skepticism, it will color your experience.

2. Find a group sound bath, and take your yoga mat with you so you can lie down comfortably. If you don't have a yoga mat, lying on a thick blanket works as well, Dusatko said. Try going to a sound bath focused on bowls and also one focused on gongs to see what you like best. You may find you prefer the sound of gongs more than a sound bath (some sound baths also incorporate gongs).

3. Don't give up after attending one session. Try several different places to experience different styles of sound baths. (According to Dusatko, there are a few contraindications regarding sound baths. For example, it is not advisable to go to one in the early stages of pregnancy or soon after an operation.)

4. If you are looking for extreme relaxation and stress reduction, Dusatko recommends looking for a vibrational sound therapy practitioner and experiencing a one-on-one session with Himalayan singing bowls on the body.

5. If you do decide to try an online sound bath, make sure to wear good-quality headphones or earbuds or have high-quality speakers to get the most benefit.

6 If you're buying a singing bowl, find a reputable shop that sells them in-store so you can test them out. Keep in mind that your current state of mind might attract you to certain tones or the feeling you get when you play a specific one.

7 Finally, keep experimenting if you like how you feel when you engage with sound bowls. How you experience certain tones can change based on what you're going through in your life.

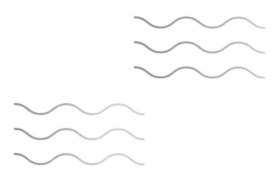

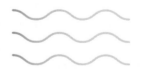

38

Get Lost in a Good Story

As of May 2022, there were more than two billion podcasts and forty-eight million episodes, according to PodcastHosting.org. More than half (55 percent) of the U.S. population listens to a podcast each month with almost a quarter (24 percent) listening to them weekly.

For many, like Shannan Hofman Bunting and Tracy Seglin, listening to podcasts regularly has become an important part of their entertainment diet, serves as a helpful distraction and a way to focus and, yes, even calms them in their own way.

It might be the storytelling that appeals to most people—similar to how some of us experienced listening to the radio or being read to by a parent or caregiver when we were younger. That's how Seglin, a freelance writer and podcast enthusiast, describes one of the reasons she loves tuning in to podcasts. There is something familiar and comforting about listening to podcasts to gather information or be entertained. She admits that she didn't actively seek out podcasts with the intention of them calming her, but there are some she is drawn to because they have a calming effect. She compares listening to podcasts to being a bit like theater for the mind.

Listening to a podcast might be a better alternative than listening to an audiobook because podcasts are short and you can hear a whole story within a bite-sized chunk of time rather than having to commit to several hours of listening.

One study published in the journal *Nature* concluded that listening to narrative stories (much like podcasts) can stimulate multiple parts of your brain. Some may experience an adrenaline rush from listening to true crime podcasts or a boost in endorphins from tuning in to a comedy podcast, for example.

True crime podcasts as relaxing? While Seglin listens to a wide range of genres, from true crime to poetry, depending on her mood, she does love them for the escapism they provide. "I would describe them as candy," she explained, "a great distraction like a summer beach read."

The reason might be thanks to how our brains interpret suspense. Hannah Malach, who wrote an article for *Good Housekeeping*, asked materials scientist and engineer Titi Shodiya, who hosts the podcast *Dope Labs* alongside molecular biologist Zakiya Whatley, for some insights into how listening to different types of podcasts can affect your brain. For those who love things that are more stimulating, there is a scientific reason the genre appeals to some listeners.

"Your brain interprets particularly suspenseful information through the medulla oblongata, which produces adrenaline. This stress-inducing chemical triggers your 'fight or flight' response. The rush you might get from listening to true crime also activates your pituitary gland, releasing endorphins. Endorphins affect your brain similarly to opioids, meaning they can be slightly addictive. This type of podcast can also lead to the production of dopamine and serotonin," Malach wrote. "Dopamine and serotonin are both feel-good chemicals, so it gives you the feeling of 'I'm terrified—but I like it,'" explained Shodiya.

Another reason Seglin loves true crime podcasts is they allow her to get lost in a story, and that can be calming. "If you're feeling stress in your life," Seglin told me, "there's something to be said about how distraction can be calming. Like finding out about a crime that is not related to your actual life."

Listening to podcasts is a welcome distraction from what's going on in the world and even lets you focus. While Bunting admits podcasts are an intrinsic part of her day, she loves listening to the story-focused ones like *Serial* and *This American Life*.

If Bunting needs to be in a car for a lengthy amount of time, she plots out which podcasts to listen to because they'll make the time pass more quickly.

Bunting also loves listening to story podcasts while walking or running. "Having to concentrate on the stories takes me out of my own head; otherwise I would be making to-do lists and sending myself emails to remember things rather than enjoying walking or exercising," she told me.

"Listening to podcasts is a great escape for me," Bunting

added. "And if it gets me to walk more, that is a double bonus—mental and physical wellness!"

There is yet another reason podcasts play an important role in Seglin's life. She loves them so much that she created a podcast club so she could meet with others to discuss podcasts they enjoy listening to. "We meet once a month, and it's just like a book club where someone picks a podcast," she explained. "It can be a stand-alone episode, or it could be a whole series."

About thirteen people are part of the group, but in reality, about six to nine meet regularly. The club has become so strong that in the fall of 2021, eleven of them went on a weekend getaway to Saugatuck, Michigan, for one of their monthly get-togethers.

TRY IT

1. Before you can start listening to a podcast, you need to download a podcast player app such as Apple Podcasts, Stitcher, Google Podcasts, Spotify, or Audible (there are others). Then, use the search function to search for types of podcasts you might be interested in hearing. Type in words like *self-help*, *true crime*, *comedy*, or *gardening*, and see what pops up. Once you find a few you like, the app will offer recommendations.

2. Also, if you're not already a podcast listener, Seglin recommends starting with one of the meditation-focused podcasts since many of us are really good about consuming auditory calming through apps. She admits you can't really tune into

those while doing activities like driving or shopping, but they might be helpful when you need downtime, like before going to bed, or even when you want to start your day on a calm note.

3. Ask your friends for recommendations. Let them know what kind of stories you enjoy reading or movies you like. Do you enjoy watching the news regularly? Or watching comedy shows? Or maybe you like reading motivational books. Their recommendations might surprise you.

4. For those who love more storytelling-oriented podcasts, try *This American Life*, *Serial*, *The Moth*, and *Wait, Wait, Don't Tell Me*.

5. Create a routine around listening to a podcast. Many of them drop new episodes on a schedule. Some of my favorites would drop on Thursdays, for example, and I'd schedule a thirty-minute elliptical session at the gym just so I could listen to the new episode. Another dropped on Friday mornings, so I'd save that one for a long bath on Sunday night before starting my work week the following day.

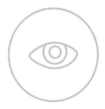

See

The question is not what you look at—but how you look and whether you see.

HENRY DAVID THOREAU

(39)

Nurturing Nature

Plants sustain us and nurture us. Like air and water, we need plants to survive. Spending time in nature can improve our mental health, but does spending time with houseplants have the same effect? Indoor houseplants don't just look good, they also play a role in human health and comfort, according to the *Journal of Environmental Science and Pollution Research*.

Thanks to the power of social media, the secret is out. Houseplants are suddenly in vogue again, and nurseries and garden centers are trying to keep up with demand, especially after the COVID-19 pandemic hit. Since we spend almost 90 percent of our time indoors, it's no surprise that what's inside our homes or workplaces is important for our health.

Millennials are helping fuel this demand, according to

Nursery Management, a trade magazine geared toward nursery and garden center owners and buyers. "Compared to previous years, the houseplant trend has interested new clientele, but the plants themselves are no longer for looks and home décor. Now, they are part of a greater focus on lifestyle and health," wrote Sierra Allen, author of the piece "The Houseplant Hype."

According to Holli Schippers, the houseplant and seasonal manager at Sunnyside Nursery in Marysville, Washington, about two-thirds of customers who visit their shop seek out air-purifying plants, and she believes it's because they want to be healthier. "What I get is, 'What can I use for air-purifying plants?' That is constant, constant, constant. People want to clean the air in their house."

Justin Hancock, head of Costa Farms' brand and consumer marketing, agrees with Schippers and added, "Millennials in particular are really interested in their wellness and that audience has created more momentum."

Plants as Therapy

In a world filled with incessant digital pings and endless screen time, caring for houseplants also serves another purpose as a form of therapy. Simply caring for a plant just a few minutes a day or once a week provides enormous benefits and offers us a sense of tranquility and wellness that we can cultivate indoors.

You don't need to live in an indoor jungle nor have a green thumb to reap the benefits. Once you find the type of houseplants you can grow successfully, you will soon discover the act of caring for plant life can be therapeutic and improve your physical and mental health and well-being.

In his book *Plants as Therapy*, Elvin McDonald shares that to nurture a plant is to satisfy an instinctive need and overcome everyday stress and anxiety in the process.

An expert in gardening, horticulture, photography, and publishing who has written more than fifty books, he shares a gentle moment in the book where he is wiping down the leaves of his palm plant. "The only way to clean it is to wipe one leaf at a time on both sides with damp paper toweling or a soft cotton cloth." He continues the process of general maintenance by cutting off fronds that are dead or dying. "As I tackle each phase of this bathing and grooming, my mind is at first occupied with what I am doing, but the repetitive parts quickly lull my mind into a sort of idling state. The end result is that the palm looks as fresh and healthy as those I've seen in the tropics after a refreshing shower, and that I have shifted my head out of high gear to a speed much more conducive to clear thinking and greater productivity."

Including some houseplants in your indoor space can help you lower your blood pressure and improve your memory and concentration. Consider how you feel when you notice a houseplant's flowers, a succulent's leaves, or a pretty pot.

Having a plant on your desk or in your home has been shown to lower stress levels and boost productivity. Results from a research study suggest that active interaction with indoor plants can reduce physiological and psychological stress compared with mental work. As part of the study, the researchers divided twenty-four men in their midtwenties into two groups to compare the differences in physiological responses to a computer task and a plant-related task. One group was tasked with transplanting an indoor plant, whereas the second group worked on a computer task. Afterward, each subject switched activities. Results showed that the subjects felt more comfortable, soothed, and natural after the transplanting task than after the computer task.

The obvious suggestion when life gets overwhelming is to take some time off, go on vacation, or work less. But if none of those is a viable option, houseplants are a natural alternative to taking a little break in the day. "They can help us get through a tough day, a lonely night, or a long period of anxiety," McDonald wrote. "When you're on top of the world, having plants can make life even sweeter, and when you come down, they'll be a support to you."

He added, "Plant therapy requires no prescription. It can be refilled as often as you feel the need. Addiction to gardening, indoors or outdoors, one plant or a thousand, is a desirable state."

--- TRY IT ---

For those who are ready to flex their green thumb muscles and get started, perhaps the first thing to consider is what you want to avoid: having more plants than you have time or energy to care for properly. "Grooming the right number of plants can be highly therapeutic; having too many plants with dead leaves and flowers mixed among the dusty, soot-covered growth, can of itself be depressing," McDonald noted.

Once you've decided you are ready, here are things to keep in mind:

1. Do you have direct natural light reaching the windowsill, tabletop, floor, or space to be occupied by the plant? You'll want to know where your source of light is and how much you have so you can choose a plant that will thrive in that light environment.

2. No direct sun? If not, is the natural sunlight bright enough to read? If not, you may want to choose low-light loving plants, or you'll need to supplement your space with artificial lights. Keep in mind, there are many houseplants that will thrive in low-light situations while others need a healthy dose of proper light.

3. Before heading to adopt your first houseplant, note the temperature range your plant will experience in the space as well as the humidity.

4. Armed with information on your lighting, temperature, and humidity, head to a nursery or garden center where you can ask what types of plants would do well in your space based on what you like and if you have pets or small children (some houseplants can be harmful to pets or small children if they're bothered). Do you prefer succulents or pretty foliage? Does the design of the planter make you smile? Do you want something hanging, or can the plant rest on a countertop or desk? Do you want it to flower? Based on the recommendations you're provided, you may want to consider the plant that requires the lowest maintenance to start. After you get the hang of caring for your initial plant, you can graduate by adding more.

5 If you want to try your hand at growing seeds or plants from cuttings shared from a friend or neighbor, some of the easiest plants to grow from seeds indoors are coleus, basil (the herb we eat), impatiens, and morning glory. If you have friends with houseplants, ask if you can get a cutting of their pothos, coleus, begonia, geranium, African violet, impatiens, or philodendron as all of these are relatively easy to grow from cuttings as long as there are root nodes on the stem right below the leaf or branch junctures.

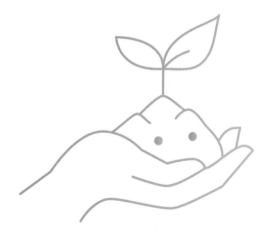

40

Chase the Light

My friend Jason Patterson once admitted that upon waking in the morning, he immediately walks directly to his living room's window, the one facing south. He opens the blinds and stands there for a few minutes. While he didn't realize why he did this, he knew that it made him feel good.

It's easy for us to fall into doldrums when it's dark outside during the winter months, especially for those of us who live in colder climates. Some of us experience seasonal affective disorder (SAD), a type of depression that occurs during the late fall and early winter and often ends by spring or early summer. Researchers are unsure of the exact cause of SAD, but research points to lack of light as the main contributor.

Bottom line: exposure to light can help.

When we're exposed to sunlight, it stimulates the hypo-thalamus, the part of the brain that helps control our circadian rhythm, which is the body's internal twenty-four-hour sleep-wake clock. When we don't get enough light, it throws off our circadian rhythms, and this can cause our brains to produce too much of the sleep hormone melatonin and to release less serotonin, the feel-good brain chemical that affects mood. This chemical imbalance is what makes us feel low and lethargic.

"SAD is not a minor condition, but because people typically experience it only during certain months, they don't see it as a serious issue. However, it is imperative to treat," said Dr. Paolo Cassano, a psychiatrist who specializes in low-level light therapy at Harvard-affiliated Massachusetts General Hospital.

Do You Suffer from SAD?

According to Harvard Health Publishing (HHP), people formally diagnosed with SAD must meet the criteria for major depressive episodes coinciding with the fall and winter months for at least two years. Here are some common symptoms of a major depressive episode associated with SAD:

* feeling hopeless or worthless
* losing interest in activities you once enjoyed
* having problems with sleep
* experiencing changes in your appetite or weight
* feeling sluggish or agitated

Since one of the ways to combat depression symptoms like those caused by SAD and improve your general mood during the cold and dark winter months is to increase exposure to light, spending time outdoors when sunlight is available is advised. Fifteen to thirty minutes of exposure to daylight provides the "awake and alert" signal our bodies need to properly regulate our hormones and circadian rhythms. For many SAD sufferers, spending as much time outdoors as possible is a natural approach.

It's understandable that some people are reluctant to go outside when it's cold and dark in the mornings. If it's safe to go outdoors, consider investing in a good pair of boots, snow pants, and a warm jacket to enjoy longer outdoor exposure once that sun comes out. Warm gloves and thick wool socks can help too.

If it's unsafe to get outdoors because of inclement weather or you have a job or family obligations that prevent you from getting outside in the morning, take advantage of any sunlight by opening the window shades in your home. In some cases, more natural sunlight in your home might be enough to treat mild cases of SAD.

When natural sunlight isn't an option, as is the case often in northern states during the winter months, phototherapy, or bright light therapy, might be a good option.

Light therapy uses light boxes that produce a bright white light. The brain recognizes the artificial light like natural sunlight. "Even if you don't yet have the clinical signs and symptoms of SAD, using light therapy during the winter may help prevent it," said Cassano in the HHP article.

To use light therapy or phototherapy, you need a light therapy lamp. A prescription isn't necessary to buy one, but it's recommended you ask your primary care provider, psychiatrist, or psychologist to make sure it's right for you, the Cleveland Clinic recommends.

It's best to be under the care of a health professional while using light therapy. While it's always a good idea to talk to a doctor or health professional before starting light therapy, it's especially important if you have any concerns about how light therapy may affect you.

—————————————— TRY IT ——————————————

Here's how to choose the right light therapy lamp for you.

1. Light therapy lamps have white fluorescent light tubes covered with a plastic screen to block ultraviolet rays, and the light is about twenty times brighter than regular indoor light. The lamps are specially designed to provide bright, blue-rich light, which can help provide the stimulus our bodies require in the mornings.

2. The intensity of the light, how long you use it, and the time of day you use the lamp are all important to keep in mind to increase its effectiveness. According to the Mayo Clinic, the intensity of the light box is recorded in lux, which is a measure of the amount of light you receive. For SAD, the typical recommendation is to use a 10,000-lux light box at a distance of about sixteen to twenty-four inches (forty-one to sixty-one centimeters) from your face.

3. If you're using a 10,000-lux light box, light therapy typically

involves daily sessions of about fifteen to thirty minutes. If you're using a lower-intensity light box, such as 2,500 lux, you may need to use it for longer sessions. For context, a bright, sunny day is 50,000 lux or more, according to HHP. Also, try to get some light time before 10:00 a.m., and avoid using a light box in the afternoon or evening because bright, blue-rich light can be very disruptive at night or cause insomnia. "As days become longer and sunnier, you will use light therapy less often, or may even stop during the spring and summer except for the occasional cloudy weeks," said Cassano.

4 Buyers should be aware there are no regulations for manufacturers marketing their lamps as beneficial to those suffering from SAD, which is why it's recommended you seek the advice of a professional. For example, some people think fluorescent light bulbs can do the trick, and while some might, many often provide only a small portion of the natural-light spectrum and suffer from flicker, which can cause headaches and eyestrain.

5 The lamps needn't be directly in the line of sight to receive the benefits, although they won't do any good if they're across the room. Using a light therapy lamp is one of the few things you can do while multitasking. Use it while making breakfast, reading, or doing other things to prepare for your day. Some choose to have their lamp off to the side of their computer monitor in the morning so they don't have to squint while working but can still get their morning fix.

6. Most people find benefits to using a light therapy lamp for SAD and notice those benefits as quickly as a few days after using it or up to two weeks. While light therapy is safe and well-tolerated by most users, according to the Cleveland Clinic, there are side effects for some users, including eyestrain, fatigue, headaches, insomnia, and irritability, and those who have diabetes or a retina condition, take some medications, or have bipolar disorder might want to avoid light therapy.

41

Slow Reading

Slow reading invites the reader to enjoy the act of reading. It can't be hurried, and one cannot multitask while slow reading.

"Digital technology is typically used to make life more efficient, but to some extent reading will be at odds with efficiency," John Miedema, author of *Slow Reading*, wrote. "Reading takes up time, and it has the power to conjure us away from the present moment. It speaks to inner faculties not always easily processed with the frame of our daily routine. It makes us think. Reading and slowness go hand in hand. It has always been a target for those who would have us more productive."

But slow reading isn't only about the pace at which you read. It's about reading with intention and allowing yourself the opportunity to see and read each word and sentence.

Growing up, Ellen Lambert considered reading a refuge. Today, Lambert, a former high school English teacher at the Dalton School in New York City who earned her PhD from Yale, continues to read for pleasure and leads the Slow Reading book group at the White Plains Public Library in White Plains, New York.

Lambert likens the idea of slow reading to slow food. "As with slow food, you want to slow down and savor it," Lambert told me. "Bypass the fast-food approach and take the time to do the real thing. You may find yourself coming to love the experience."

The former teacher in Lambert understands why some people don't love to read. Part of the challenge is that reading may have been taught to you in a way that is deadening. As an example, she says a teacher may ask a student to share three character traits in the book they are reading and being graded on. What happens is the student will hunt around for character traits, completely missing the emotional involvement that comes from slow reading.

In this scenario, one she feels is all too common, reading is not pleasurable, and students don't enjoy it. "It's an exercise," she said of the reading experience. "Or they're mining the work for an assigned essay. I look at the kind of stuff that kids are asked to do, and they're never asked to connect the work to their life."

When Lambert was going through a particularly challenging part of her life, she'd escape in a book. Reading became cathartic. She uses the example of a woman who might be going through a miserable or failed marriage. One would think she might not want to read a book with a character dealing with a miserable marriage, but in fact, reading a book like this may make her feel like she's not alone. Reading a story like this might allow her the opportunity to wonder what the main character is going to do next or how she's going to resolve a situation.

In his book, Miedema recognizes that even those who find great pleasure in reading might struggle to find the time to practice the activity. "It seems odd that a pleasurable activity would be on the decline," Miedema admitted. "Perhaps it does not seem so odd if we consider that reading requires an investment of inner resources that people may be less willing to make. Like cooking a good meal or nurturing a relationship, and unlike fast food or too much television, reading is one of those cardinal pleasures that require effort upfront but leaves the reader feeling more energized afterward. This is another reason that reading is at risk in every generation, but especially in the digital age. Our attention can only manage so many stimuli. With the endless stream of information fed to us in modern life, our attention is compromised. The Web was supposed to make information more manageable, but in fact it displaces time and attention we might spend really savoring a good read."

While it may be easy to blame digital technology as the main culprit, Miedema points to our weakness for speed and our attempts to attend to too many things at once as the true villains in this story. The reality is one truly cannot multitask when they're slow reading, and we must dedicate time for the activity. Like slow cooking requires focus and intention, slow reading requires you to immerse yourself in the experience and tune everything else out.

While reading is a solo activity, Lambert highly recommends finding and engaging with a local book club. Although she's retired now, her love and passion for slow reading haven't slowed down. To encourage slow reading and discussion, Lambert leads the Slow Reading book group at the White Plains Public Library, which is designed to foster close, attentive reading and discussion of great works of literature—both short stories and novels. The group meets every two weeks.

Lambert loves to read at night as she's preparing to go to bed. Her book is next to her bed so it's ready for her. She looks forward to that moment because once she gets under the covers, she feels like the weight of whatever she's been doing during the day is lifted. And then she picks up the book and can let everything else go. Sometimes she has a cup of tea by her side, but it's not an essential part of her slow reading experience. To her, it's like visiting with a friend through the characters and stories she's about to read.

"We cannot accelerate our lives indefinitely," Miedema wrote. "At some point, we have to slow down to get a handle on our information. Slow reading represents balance."

—————————————— TRY IT ——————————————

1 Consider the types of books you like to read, and don't be ashamed of what you enjoy. This isn't about impressing someone else with what you're reading or forcing yourself to read something because you think you should. If you like heartthrob romance novels, read those. Prefer getting lost in

science fiction or thrillers? Put those next to your bedside or wherever you plan to read.

2. Find your "book nook" and create a pleasing environment so once you're ready to read, you don't have any distractions and you're surrounded by things that will allow you to enjoy the reading experience. Does a soft blanket help? Or a coaster to set your hot cup of tea on or a small side table for a glass of wine?

3. If you're the kind of person who loves to go a bit deeper into your books or discover new books to read through others, Lambert highly recommends finding a book club or book group so you can engage in meaningful discussions around books.

4. Engage all your senses when you're reading. Light a candle, pour yourself a drink, wrap yourself up in a blanket, let your fingers hold a physical book and turn the pages, or write little notes in the margins. If it's not too distracting, place some calming music in the background.

5. Create a ritual or habit around your slow reading experience. If evenings right before you go to bed are the best time to enjoy uninterrupted reading, make that your reading time. If early morning before your day begins is better, that's fine too. Having a set time will allow you to look forward to that experience.

Living in Color

C olor is strongly attached to our emotions. From the time we're born, we can identify color contrasts, and by the time we are two or three months old, most of us can detect actual colors.

As we mature, we start to attach certain thoughts, feelings, and emotions to colors based on how those colors are introduced to us, according to Leatrice Eiseman, a color specialist whose expertise is recognized worldwide as the executive director of the Pantone Color Institute. Often, nature's colors tend to be favored thanks to how they were presented to us when we were younger by parents or caregivers.

"'Look at the beautiful blue sky,'" Eiseman offered as an example of a possible interaction between a child and an adult. "'What a clear day. We can go outside and go for a walk or you can play outside.' These are all the good things you attach to the thought of a blue sky. It's not a rainy, dreary day. The same thing would be true for yellow sunshine."

We start to show a preference for certain colors, like blue in this example, because we associate the color with good things or things we enjoy. We may be drawn to wearing the color blue on days we want to feel calmer or paint our living room a shade of blue to remind us of days at the beach on vacation.

That's not to say the color blue is everyone's favorite calm color. Perhaps a child's first tricycle was powder blue and the child fell off their bike and broke a bone and couldn't play with their friends as a result. In this case, the child may develop a negative association with the color blue.

Some may find red alarming and associate it with danger and blood, while others might be drawn to the color because it signifies energy and power.

"From the beginning of time, cave people knew that fire could warm you. It could cook your food but it could also burn your skin," Eiseman explained. "So you have all of these elements that are attached to the color red. But the primary reason is you have to pay attention to it. It's nature's biggest signal color. And so the physiological then becomes tied to the emotional and psychological."

Most of us don't consciously pay attention to the colors in our lives. We unconsciously gravitate toward certain colors because of how they make us feel. This is why it's important to identify which colors make us feel good.

Worth noting is choosing colors that calm us, or the use of color psychology, is different from color therapy, or chromotherapy. Chromotherapy is a form of therapy that uses color and light to treat certain mental and physical health conditions, and its origins date back to the ancient Egyptians. Dr. Somia Gul notes chromotherapy triggers specific points in our body and relieves various ailments in her research published in the *American Research Journal of Pharmacy*, so if this is of interest, check out chromotherapy.

Like chromotherapy, color psychology isn't new.

In a 2015 review, Andrew J. Elliot wrote in *Frontiers in Psychology* that researchers found theorizing on color and psychological functioning has been present since Goethe penned his *Theory of Colors* in 1810, in which he linked color categories (e.g., the "plus" colors of yellow, red-yellow, yellow-red) to emotional responding (e.g., warmth, excitement). While a fair amount of research has been done that shows considerable promise on color and psychological functioning, Elliot feels more theoretical and empirical work needs to be done.

Still, for those of us who love color and try to incorporate it into our lives because certain colors make us feel a certain way, there is much to appreciate about the benefits of color on our psyche.

While more research can be done on the benefits of color on our well-being, there is no doubt we react to colors, and they affect our emotions. It's worth taking the time to explore how colors affect you and bring in more of those you find calming.

———————————————— TRY IT ————————————————

If you're trying to figure out which colors will bring more calm into your life, Eiseman offers these suggestions to get started:

1. Come up with a mood that you're trying to impart.

2. If you're trying to bring in a more relaxed state of mind, close your eyes and think of a time or place where you were happy, relaxed, or calm. Were you curled up with a cup of hot coffee and a good book with a warm blanket wrapped around your lap? Is there a fireplace in the background? Are you eating a home-cooked meal lovingly prepared by your grandmother? Or hiking through the woods with your dog? Or perhaps you are walking along a sandy white beach with a blue sky and glistening blue water as far as the eye can see. Maybe you're in a dark club listening to live jazz musicians.

3. Scan that visual in your mind, and notice the colors. Are you comforted by the warm browns of the coffee or blanket? Or the green leaves on the trees along a nature walk? Or the white-gray sand and light blue sky at the beach? Or maybe you feel the dark lounge atmosphere of a jazz club is soothing.

4. Take a deep breath, and consider how those colors make you feel.

5. Once you determine which colors make you feel calmer and relaxed, try to introduce more of those into your life, and remove others that make you feel anxious. For example, I love

the color blue and have intentionally added more blue-toned clothing to my wardrobe because it gets me out of reaching for my black clothes as a default and it makes me feel better. Similarly, I'm ditching black dress boots for my maroon Doc Martens or grabbing my mustard-yellow handbag instead of my black leather bag. See a pattern? For me, it's easy to reach for black. But by slowly adding colors I love and that make me happy into my daily wardrobe choices, I'm also adding calm without realizing it.

6. A big way to introduce color into your life is by painting the interior walls of your house. But Eiseman points out that many people are nervous when choosing a paint color for walls. It's not something they change every day, and they want to make sure they get it right. Still, she said, it's just a can of paint. Walls can be repainted. "It shouldn't be a source of trauma."

7. She encourages people to channel their inner child who took great delight in taking a box of crayons and scribbling or coloring outside the lines. Experiment! You may realize a color you wouldn't have considered is exactly the color that works for you and brings you joy.

8. Resist the urge to choose a color that might satisfy someone else, something, Eiseman said, we do more often than we think. "As people grow older, they become more aware of those who surround them and the criticism that they might get from choosing a particular color."

⑨ There is more to color than the paint on our walls. People who love high design gravitate toward using products infused with colors that make them feel better, according to Eiseman. When I was in the market for a laptop, I could have defaulted with the silver case. A rose-gold one was an option, although it cost $100 more. I bought the rose-gold case and have never once regretted the additional cost because every time I see my laptop or reach to use it, the color makes me happy. It's such a utilitarian product, but there is no reason it can't be pretty.

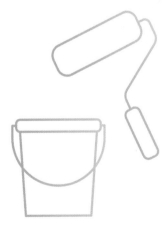

Art for Art's Sake

When we walk into an art museum, it seems we're always rushed. We usually make plans to visit one as a destination, as a weekend excursion with friends or to see a particular exhibit. And due to the cost to visit most of them, we try to maximize our time by rushing through as many rooms as possible, making it hard to really "see" anything.

All of which is a shame because looking at art is beneficial to our well-being.

Oshin Vartanian, an expert on the neuroscience of aesthetics and creativity at the University of Toronto, explored the different ways people observe and appreciate art on a neurological level. In a Q&A published in *U of T News*, Vartanian found that certain areas of the brain involved in processing emotion and those that activate our pleasure and reward systems are being engaged. "We also found that the brain's default mode network—the area associated with internally-oriented thinking like daydreaming, thinking about the future or retrieving memories—is also activated," he shared. "So what's happening is that areas associated with more contemplative responses are being triggered automatically when people view art even if they don't have instructions to judge or think about it critically."

According to Vartanian, one area actively engaged while viewing art is the interior insula, which historically has been associated with experiencing pain. "Many early studies of the brain found that this area would be activated when viewing paintings and even sculpture, which didn't make immediate sense because we tend to associate viewing artworks with some form of pleasure," he explained. "However, what a lot of recent studies have found is that this area is also responsible for experiencing pleasant emotions, especially ones that have a visceral aspect to them. Another area that's engaged when viewing art is the putamen. This area is part of the basal ganglia, an important system in the brain for the experience of reward, among other things."

Phyl Terry isn't surprised by art's power to activate our brains in different ways. He founded Slow Art Day to remind us to slow down, look at a painting, and allow ourselves time to fully take in the work. To really *see* it.

He invites people to use the dedicated day celebrated annually in April to discover that you can have a relationship to art and be part of the experience, even if you think you know nothing about art.

Terry was CEO of a customer experience consulting firm, working with clients like Google and Apple and helping them think about design, strategy, and customer experiences. He came to love art, both because he thought it was great inspiration for design in any field, including business, and also for its own sake. "It's a fundamental impulse of the human species to create and participate in art," Terry told me.

Maggie Levine is drawn to abstract art, and while she admits she's not sure she'd use the term *calming* to explain her experience of looking at abstract pieces, she does like the feeling of being taken out of her own neuroses. Instead, she prefers to use the verb *engaged*.

"I love losing myself in the repetition of all of these shapes," Levine told me. "I like the kinds of associations and responses that come up in my brain."

Levine prefers abstract art to other types, like conceptual art, because "it's devoid of clear meanings so that I can just enjoy the different languages that are available to painters," she explained.

The texture of abstract art appeals to her too, not so much because it calms her when she looks at the work of these "painterly painters," as she calls them, but it's where her appreciation senses start to ding.

For those wondering how to get started, Slow Art Day can help. You don't need a degree in art history to appreciate what art brings into your life. Nor do you need any art experience to walk into a museum and look at a piece of art. You also don't need to have a lot of money or to become a collector. Art is and should be available to anyone.

Despite the power viewing art can have on our lives, personally and professionally, Terry knows the majority of American people do not go to art museums, and he hopes Slow Art Day changes that reality. "They find [art museums] intimidating, boring, some combination of things, not connected to it," he said, ticking off excuses like a checklist.

Many museums are opening their doors to the communities they serve by offering free museum days throughout the year. Some are even creating programs to cater specifically to the health and well-being of different populations, from young school-aged children to those with Alzheimer's disease or dementia. In a report published by the Research Centre for Museums and Galleries, School of Museum Studies at the University of Leicester, titled "Mind, Body, Spirit: How Museums Impact Health and Wellbeing," the authors note there is a growing body of museums addressing community health and well-being, offering health promotion and education, and tackling health inequalities. "Many of these projects are innovative or experimental, stimulating new ways of using collections or addressing specific themes, groups or issues," the authors wrote.

One of those programs was Meet Me at MoMA, the New York Museum of Modern Art's program for people in the early stages of dementia or Alzheimer's disease and their caregivers, which was offered between 2007 and 2014. "During this time, MoMA staff expanded on the success of the museum's existing education programs for individuals with dementia and their care partners through the development of training resources intended for use by arts and health professionals on how to make art accessible to people with dementia using MoMA's teaching methodologies and approach."

No matter your age, taking the time to experience art can be transformative. Terry and Levine want people to give art a chance. Levine's Substack newsletter called ARTWRITE is a way for her to explore the creative process through a blend of personal narrative and interviews with visual artists. "Instead of reviewing or analyzing art, each issue groups artists around a theme such as memory or intention," she shared on her professional website page. "It's different from most art writing because it's accessible and never critical."

But Levine and Terry insist the type of art doesn't matter. Look at different pieces, and see what you're drawn to. It could be contemporary art, classic, ancient, impressionist, abstract expressionist, you name it; just identify any single piece of art, and look at it for at least ten minutes.

"The first minute will be slow, and they will experience it slow," Terry explained. He joked the name "Slow Art Day" has a branding problem because people think if watching paint dry is a bummer, try asking them to watch dry paint for a long time.

"But we know that once people sit down and look, and if they allow themselves to slow down, [it] will blow their minds," Terry said. "They will build a relationship and they will include themselves in the art experience."

The problem is most people, if they go to a museum at all, look at a piece of art for about ten seconds, and that is not only not transformative, it is deadening. They seem to look at everything and see nothing. And then they don't want to return because they're exhausted from trying to see it all.

In the prelude of *Looking at Mindfulness: Twenty-Five Paintings to Change the Way You Live*, author Christophe André references Rembrandt's *Philosopher in Meditation* painting and notes that the first thing most of us see is the intense yellow light of the winter sun outside a window. Then he leads us through the rest of the painting— the old man sitting motionless, having turned away from his table, and the book he was studying. The author is wondering what he's thinking. Is he resting? Meditating? He continues by asking the reader questions about where our eyes might land next and what we might be drawn to.

"This is the genius of Rembrandt, who leads us on a visual journey through all the dimensions," André wrote.

This experience is available to all of us. When we give ourselves permission to look at a piece of art for more than a mere few seconds, we're able to take in the piece and see things that are less obvious than from an immediate or tertiary glance. We can really experience it, get to know it, let it sit with us, and see how we feel about it. What it means to us. How it might reflect what we're dealing with at any given moment.

─────────────── TRY IT ───────────────

1. Set aside a date to visit a museum near you on your own. If cost is an issue, find one to visit during its free museum days—almost all museums offer at least one day or evening a month for residents to visit for free. Others request a modest

donation. Some also offer discounts for students, teachers, members of the military, or seniors.

2 Rather than be tempted to rush through each of the galleries, limit yourself to one or two galleries. Once you're in the first one, find one painting or piece you're drawn to, and stay with it for at least ten minutes. Allow yourself a longer period if you're so inclined.

3 If you want something more formal or organized, add Slow Art Day to your calendar, and see if your local museum is participating. The day lands every year on the first Saturday in April.

4 Don't forget that art is everywhere if you pause long enough to notice it. It can be in the form of public art, a mural beneath a viaduct, sculptures in a park, or art adorning the walls of your favorite coffee shop.

5 Finally, make it a point to visit a new museum or gallery regularly, whether that means once a month or once a quarter. You may think you are drawn to one type of art only to discover you like other types too.

44

Inside the Lines

In 2016, Jordan Gaines Lewis, a science writer and neuro-science PhD student at Penn State College of Medicine at the time, admitted in an article for *New York* magazine's The Cut that she caved and bought herself a coloring book.

A few nights a week, she would curl up on the couch with her ever-growing collection of colored pencils, tune in to the latest episode of *Serial*, and scribble away at mandalas and Harry Potters.

Like many busy people, Gaines Lewis was surprised at her attraction to something so not in her wheelhouse. Coloring within the lines of a mandala or other illustrations doesn't require a lot of brain power. You're not producing anything original. You're not creating a "piece of art," per se.

But here's the thing. If we enjoy doing something, and it brings us some levity in an otherwise hellish day, or we look forward to the experience for the way it makes us feel calmer, must we assign some currency to it? Must everything we do be in the interest of working toward a goal, to make something or to commodify it?

Nathalie Kunin doesn't think so. The consultant by day received a paint-by-numbers kit from her mom that was meant as a gag gift—a flower in a water jug illustration. "I kind of knew vaguely, obviously, what paint by numbers was, but it was rolled up in a tube and it was very pretty," she told me. She rolled it out, and she and her husband began doing it together, side by side. Once they started coloring in the design using the paints provided, they admitted the experience was really fun and did another few together, eventually deciding to do their own. To accommodate their growing interest, they transformed their Los Angeles kitchen into a mini art studio. She draped an art cloth a friend gave her as a birthday gift over her kitchen table, and now she and her husband sit across from each other, overlooking their beautiful backyard, as they work on their masterpieces. Her kitchen, bathed in natural light, equipped with water and their dipping brushes, has become their place of refuge. Sometimes they'll sit together without speaking and just work on their canvases, sometimes they'll chitchat, sometimes they'll listen to music or a podcast. Sometimes they'll work on their pieces separately.

How often are they drawn to work on their respective canvases?

"Certainly once a day, but often even more than once a day," Kunin said. "Just for ten or fifteen minutes."

Kunin is drawn to nature scenes while her husband tends to choose city scenes.

"It's an incredible stress reliever," Kunin admitted. She talked about how much all of it contributes to the calm she feels when she sits down to work on her canvas, everything from the theme of the illustration to the colors of the paint to feeling the brush in her hand as she's painting. "The painting," she added, "is very soothing, very cathartic."

She paints while she's having an important or serious phone call, but her husband doesn't like to work while painting. He prefers to listen to music or a podcast and get into the moment. "Sometimes before he comes up to bed, if I'm already upstairs, he'll paint for fifteen minutes," Kunin noted. "I think it decompresses him."

One of the reasons coloring books or paint-by-numbers kits are so appealing to many is that they don't require any prior experience or expertise. There is no right or wrong way to color within or even outside the lines of a coloring book or to brush paint over a shape with a number on it. And since it requires some concentration and repetition, it can be particularly meditative.

"It's very focused but you're not making any big decisions," Kunin explained as one of the reasons this activity appeals to her and why she finds it so calming. "It's almost like occupational therapy, in the sense that it's very soothing. It's the process. And you may love the outcome."

In a study published in *Art Therapy*, available to members through the American Art Therapy Association, authors Nancy A. Curry and Tim Kasser noted the basic idea of coloring therapy, which includes activities like coloring mandalas, is that when individuals color complex geometric forms, they are provided an opportunity to suspend their "inner dialogue" and to deeply engage in an activity that removes them from the flow of negative thoughts and emotions that can sometimes dominate their lives.

The study had participants color a mandala or a plaid design or draw whatever they liked using colors on a blank page. What the authors discovered is having something to color in a structured way (like an illustration) helped soothe anxiety, whereas allowing participants the option of doing whatever they wanted on a blank page may have contributed to creating anxiety (or at least didn't help reduce anxiety).

"If anxiety is a type of inner chaos, it seems likely that a structured activity such as coloring a predetermined, somewhat complex design would help to organize that chaos," the authors wrote. "In contrast, participants in the freeform condition had to find their own way to structure their experience for 20 minutes, and this may either have been anxiety-inducing itself or have failed to help them reduce their anxiety."

Other reasons people are drawn to coloring to help calm their body and mind? It's an analog hobby, it's relatively affordable, and anyone who can hold a brush or coloring pencil can do it, whether it's a young child just learning to grasp a pencil or an adult who has the dexterity to hold a paintbrush.

Johanna Basford, an illustrator whose first book, *Secret Garden*, sold nearly 1.5 million copies, said in an interview, "I think there's something quite charming and nostalgic about coloring in. And chances are the last time you picked up pens or pencils you didn't have a mortgage or like a really horrible boss or anything. So yeah, it's just a really nice way to be creative. You don't have to sit down with a blank sheet of paper or, you know, have that scary moment of thinking, 'What can I draw?' The outlines are already there for you, so it's just something that you can do quietly for a couple of hours that, you know, is handheld and analog and quiet."

Kunin and her husband have completed two dozen pieces *each* since they started their hobby, and if you're wondering where those completed masterpieces are today, a dozen are hanging proudly and prominently in their dining room. She originally asked her husband to keep them within that one room, but she admits some have migrated into other rooms. A few hang in her son's bedroom while he's away at college, and a couple are in their bathroom. "I might not have framed as many, but my husband loves looking at them," she added. "I do it more for the process."

TRY IT

1. If you have some room in your house to lay out a canvas, go online and see if you can find a design you're drawn to. Each paint-by-number kit comes with its own paints, so you don't have to worry about having to buy more equipment. Some come with a brush, while others offer it as an add-on when you buy a kit.

2. If you don't have space in your home or need something

more portable, look at coloring books. Other than the book, if you don't already own colored pencils, you might have to invest in a box, but usually the cost is minimal and they last a long time.

3 If you want a little sass, there are coloring books that use swear words as part of the design to color in. One customer of such a book noted in an Amazon review that she uses the book to help calm down without the need to swear. Another customer notes she turns to her swear coloring book when she's upset with someone so she can "color my feelings and let it be between myself and my higher power and speak gently to the one I'm upset with." Swear coloring books might not be for everyone, but they could be a great stress reliever if it's your cup of tea.

4 Dedicate a time of day to spend a few minutes with your work. It could be five minutes while drinking your coffee in the morning as you prepare for your day, or it could be just before you retire for the night. Having a coloring book around and nearby allows you to access it whenever you need it.

5 Some people find pleasure sharing their final pieces with others, either via a social media platform like Instagram or hanging them in their home.

6 If you're planning to have a serious conversation with a loved one, Kunin highly recommends pulling out a paint-by-number canvas and inviting your family member or friend

to paint or color with you. By focusing on something else together, she feels it can defuse the situation a bit or reduce the adrenaline feeling.

7. Finally, appreciate that the experience is more than just painting or the final product hanging on a wall. From reviewing kit options online to the anticipation of the package arriving to opening up the paint colors for the first time, Kunin said all of it gives her a rush. "Part of that is just the sheer visual," she admitted, "and then part is the anticipation of the tactile experience."

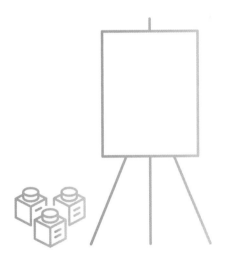

SEE

45

Dress with Less

Could you wear the same thing for one hundred days straight? And before you ask, yes, you'd be able to wash the item.

As soon as we wake up, our minds are called on to make decisions. Hit the snooze button or get out of bed? What are we going to wear? What are we going to eat? What are the plans for the day? Will I need to set aside workout clothes?

According to some estimates, we make roughly thirty-five thousand decisions a day. On the opposite side of the spectrum is the paradox of choice. When faced with too many options, we become paralyzed with indecision.

What if we pared down our options and eliminated some of those decisions? Deciding what to wear in the morning isn't usually one of the hardest decisions most of us need to make on any given day, but for some, it can make a dif-ference in how they feel.

According to Brandon Oto, a certified physician assistant in the adult ICU at UConn Health (John Dempsey Hospital), "almost any decision-making or other task requiring self-control will drain your reserves of mental energy; however, the more weighty (high stakes) or the more difficult (com-plex) the decision, the more it will cost you."

In an effort to minimize the number of decisions she needs to make throughout her day, Christy Pino of North Carolina actively seeks ways to put repetitive decisions in her life on autopilot, from creating a grocery list with standard items she uses in her household to decluttering her belongings.

When Pino stumbled on a challenge to wear the same dress for one hundred days straight and she learned the dress was from an ethical company with sustainable manufacturing methods, she was all in.

"Spending the last three months in this challenge has taught me that no one else really notices or cares what we wear," Pino admitted. "This has given me the freedom to embrace the idea that not only can I own less, but I really don't even have to be particularly creative in turning an item into different outfits. Wearing the same dress every day has given me time to focus on other things in the morning (like snug-gling with my toddler) instead of trying to figure out what my outfit will be for the day. I start off in a calmer, more confident headspace when one decision is already made."

Pino and I met because we both participated in the chal-lenge. Like her, I was drawn to the idea of minimizing my morning stress level by removing the task of figuring out what to wear—even on weekends, when I could be more casual. Could I make it one hundred days without seeing myself in something other than my dress?

Not only did I make it to one hundred days wearing one dress, but it also felt fantastic. I did my challenge over winter months so I added sweaters and scarves, but the process was cathartic in that it allowed me to view my entire wardrobe differently. First, I realized I didn't need the mountains of clothing I'd acquired over the years but barely wore. Second, having so many articles of clothing also meant I had to wade through them to decide what to wear, even though I knew I wasn't going to wear 85 percent of what was hanging in my closet. That physical clutter was causing mental clutter. I immediately started to remove items from my closet and dresser drawers and began a donation pile and consignment pile. As I was freeing up and seeing more empty space in my bedroom, it felt like I was experiencing more mental clarity too. I could physically see everything I owned and what I loved to wear more easily. I prioritized fabrics that made me feel better too. That decision paralysis from having too much stuff to review on a daily basis was lifted.

Rebecca Eby is the customer experience manager for Wool&, the company from which Pino and I bought our dresses to wear for the one-hundred-day challenge. Eby isn't surprised by how strongly women react to the dress challenge. For some, it's the first time they've taken a hard look at the amount of clothes they own, how much they spend on clothes, and the materials with which they're made.

"Many of them realize that they have so many more pieces of clothing than they need, and they prefer the simplicity of a pared down wardrobe," Eby told me. "We've heard that they fall in love with the breathability and practicality of soft merino wool, and then they begin to work on replacing many of their clothing items with more natural fibers. I think our society is so used to the prevalence of fibers like polyester that we don't realize how much we've adapted until we make the switch to natural fibers like merino. It's only then that we see how great our clothing can feel and how much simpler it is to live because of what that piece of clothing is made from."

While this activity is focused on a dress challenge, you can opt to go with fewer pieces of something else in your closet like shoes or coats. Gamifying the experience like doing a one-hundred-day challenge puts a beginning and end date on your activity, and once you see how it's affecting your life, you can decide whether you want to explore extending it to other parts of your life too.

_____ TRY IT _____

1. Think about what is motivating you to do this kind of a challenge or why paring your closet could help calm your body and mind. Slow down and really listen to your body.

2. If you're planning to pare down your closet and feel overwhelmed, some organizing experts recommend hanging every item with the hanger hook in the opposite direction. Then, when you select an item to wear, turn the hook around. At the end of the season or year, whatever hanger is still in

the opposite direction may be a strong candidate for a dona-tion or to sell. It's a faster and easier way to really see what you're drawn to and wear on a regular basis.

3   If you decide to try something like a one-hundred-day dress challenge, hang your dress in a special spot each evening to air out, Pino recommends. "Preferably somewhere between where you sleep and your closet so that you have to physically decide to bypass the dress and go put something else on when the challenge feels tough."

4   Seek out natural fibers like merino wool, linen, or cashmere, and invest in your clothes rather than getting caught up with fast fashion. You will look and feel better, the items in your wardrobe will last longer, and you won't waste money on clothing that harms the environment.

5   Enjoy the extra time in the morning not having to decide what to wear since you'll have pared down your wardrobe to the things you enjoy wearing most. Choose to use that time as you wish, whether it's to meditate, journal, or enjoy a few quiet minutes of solace with a hot cup of tea or coffee.

46

Digital Detox

As soon as we wake up, we check our phones. When driving or bicycling, we have to be on the lookout for people hunched over their mobile devices so as not to run over them. It's not unusual to see people driving and texting at the same time. At restaurants, our phones sit on the table as if on standby, even though someone we *want* to spend time with is sitting across from us.

As more of us use our smartphones and other internet-connected devices daily, our reliance on them has increased significantly. In early 2021, 31 percent of U.S. adults reported that they go online "almost constantly," up from 21 percent in 2015, according to a Pew Research Center survey conducted from January 25 to February 8, 2021. Almost half, 48 percent, admitted they go online several times a day, while only 6 percent said they go online about once a day.

Brian X. Chen noticed his online activity changed drastically during the pandemic. In a piece he wrote for the *New York Times*, he shared that before the pandemic, he was averaging about three and a half hours of screen time on his phone. Eight months later, it had nearly doubled. Ask any of your friends and family, and it's likely you'll hear a similar story—our digital devices have practically become appendages.

The problem is we think this constant connectivity can be helpful because it's keeping us connected, but the reality is that screen time is also hurting our minds and bodies. Staring at screens means we're not taking the time to see or appreciate what's around us—literally and figuratively. When we're busy looking at our phones, we may not realize we're also walking into traffic. Or not hearing our children excitedly tell us about their day. Or enjoying the walk with our dogs. It's messing with our eating habits and sleep patterns.

Maybe that's not you. Maybe you're thinking you need to check your phone or email often because of work-related communication. Fair enough, but do you have to check it around the clock? Round-the-clock monitoring of work email may be negatively affecting your mental health and leading to decreases in well-being, as one study found. Checking your email less overall leads to lower stress levels, Dr. Kostadin Kushlev, who leads the Digital Health and Happiness Lab (or Happy Tech Lab) at Georgetown University's Department of Psychology, and Dr. Elizabeth Dunn, professor in the Department of Psychology at the University of British Columbia, found in their study published in *Computers in Human Behavior*.

None of this is anecdotal. Research shows intense or frequent mobile phone usage is associated with a broad array of mental health related symptoms, behaviors, and psychological factors. In a study published in the *International Journal of Environmental Research and Public Health,* researcher Sara Thomée noted that high mobile phone use can impact sleep habits, dependency/addiction issues, and individual personality traits. "The extent to which mobile phone use interferes with the restorative functions of sleep can, of course, contribute to deteriorated health," she wrote as part of the published results. "Besides sleep being postponed, replaced, or disturbed by messages or calls at night, it is also conceivable that quantity as well as content of use can generate higher levels of psychological stress and physiological arousal. Higher levels of arousal can have a negative impact on sleep and recoveryand in other ways contribute to stress and ill health."

While the study didn't review all scenarios and the impacts of phone use such as attention, consequences for relationships, or cyberbullying, Thomée feels it is also conceivable that the time spent on devices takes time from other activities and health-related behaviors, such as physical activity, supportive social interactions, or staying on task at work or school.

Does this mean we need to ditch our phones and bring back fax machines? Hardly. Engaging in a digital detox doesn't mean we need to abandon our devices and go tech-free, but it does mean we need to better examine why we use them as we do and balance our time using them. Despite the advances our phones and computers have given us and from which we've immensely benefited, we've somehow traded away meaningful and IRL (in real life) human interaction. Texting or instant messaging gives us the illusion of connection, and it opens up the possibility of missing important nuances we get from body language and inflections.

Here's a test to see if you might be unintentionally using your phone when you don't even realize you're reaching for it: When you're waiting in line either in a drive-through or inside a coffee shop, rather than keep your phone in your pocket or purse and check out your surroundings or (gasp!) talk to someone else waiting for their drink, do you mindlessly grab it and scroll to see if you have any new emails or texts? Or when you're bored at home, rather than call a friend, go for a walk outside, or meet up with someone for a meal, do you pull up YouTube or TikTok and scroll through videos?

Using your phone to keep in touch with friends and family isn't a bad thing. Before our digital devices crept into our lives, we lost touch with some people we didn't like or whose relevance to our lives diminished over time, and that was perfectly natural, according to Daniel J. Levitin, PhD, a neuroscientist, cognitive psychologist, and author of *The Organized Mind*. Now those people, for better or for worse, can easily find us online, but most people find the pluses of being found outweigh the minuses. "We get news feeds, the equivalent of the town crier or hair salon gossip, delivered to our tablets and phones in a continuous stream," he wrote. "We can tailor those streams to give us contact with what or whom we most care about, our own personal social ticker tape. It's not a replacement for personal contact but a supplement, an easy way to stay connected to people who are far-flung and, well, just busy."

Levitin continues by admitting there might be an illusion to all this. "Social networking provides breadth but rarely depth, and in-person contact is what we crave, even if the online contact seems to take away some of that craving," he said. "In the end, the online interaction works best as a supplement, not a replacement for in-person contact."

Does this mean you need to turn off your devices if you're using your computer to work or go to school when you're actually working or studying? Of course not. In both of these cases, you need access to your computer, and you're using your devices deliberately and intentionally. It's when we default to our phones when we're bored, pull up pages on our laptops or tablets to pass time, or feel we need to be "on" twenty-four seven and responding to emails from work or posting photos on Instagram that things start to become an issue. We start feeling like we "need" to be checking email, responding to texts, or constantly updating our social media accounts lest our follower numbers take a nosedive.

It's possible to slowly remove ourselves from our digital devices. Even if we start making small changes, that time off-screen adds up, and we can "find" the time to do other things that help our overall health and well-being, whether it's spending more time with our family and friends, working out, or letting our brains take a break and do nothing at all.

─────────── TRY IT ───────────

1 SET BOUNDARIES. No one is expecting you to check your email or social media accounts as soon as you wake up or before you go to bed. Resist the urge to reach for your

phone during these times. If it helps, put your phone in another room entirely, and if you use your phone as an alarm, buy yourself an actual alarm clock to replace it.

2 **SCHEDULE TIME ON AND OFF.** Some people love to keep a schedule, so if this is you, schedule when you'll be on and when you'll be off. Ironically, there are even apps to help you! The Freedom app (which I have used myself to work on this book) allows you to block apps and websites so you can focus on whatever you're doing. If deep focus is a goal, there are also other things you can try like Focusmate. While Focusmate does require you to be online, it connects you with someone for fifty minutes at a time to focus on whatever it is you want to focus on—whether it's reading a book, cleaning your home, or whatever else you'd like to do during that time. It's a way of "coworking" but also keeping you accountable during those fifty minutes. Also, rather than just say you're going to keep to your schedule, make it more concrete by detailing how this will look for you. Will you put your phone in a drawer once you get home from work or your kids come home from school? Or can you make your table, where you eat and enjoy time with your loved ones, device-free? Or let your boss know you won't be checking or responding to emails from 7:00 p.m. to 8:00 a.m.?

3 **GO ANALOG.** We often use our phones or digital devices to replace things we used to do offline, like using a paper planner to keep our schedule or that alarm clock to wake us up. We kept a running grocery list next to the refrigerator

and did our shopping in a store. While having phones and computers has made things easier, it's also made us rely on them more. Where it makes sense, try going analog.

④ TRACK YOUR TIME. You may think you're not online as often as you are. In fact, similarly, most people don't think they eat as much as they do until they start tracking everything they put into their mouths and realize a snack here and there adds up in calories. It's the same idea with your devices. Again, there are apps to track your time, so start this week to see what your baseline is, and then try to cut that time by thirty minutes a day. Thirty minutes might be harder than you think, but if you can avoid checking your phone or emails in the morning and before you go to bed, you might hit that figure easily. The goal is to get back that control of your time and know you have the power to determine how you spend it.

⑤ DO SOMETHING ELSE. Before you reach for your phone because you're bored or "just want to quickly check something," consider the time you'd be wasting, and do something else instead. Maybe pull a cookbook from your shelf and flip through it to see if there is a recipe you want to try. Work on a jigsaw puzzle on your table. Write in your journal. Take a walk outside for fifteen minutes. Brew some tea and enjoy the silence. Consider that time a treat for yourself.

SEE

Create an Oasis

O ur homes are our private sanctuaries; home is a place where we can be ourselves, laugh, cry, make delicious meals, curl up on the couch to watch a show, or just take a break and unwind. The world outside our homes' walls can be harsh, busy, and unrelenting. But once we step inside our homes, we can let down our guard and just be. We may not be able to control what's going on outside our four walls, but inside our homes, it's a different story.

What do you see when you walk through your door?

If you want your home to reflect how you want to feel, and it's currently cluttered or messy for your taste, it may be worth reviewing your interior space and seeing what needs to go.

Even if it's not disorganized, reviewing your surroundings room by room through a self-care lens may help you see things differently.

For example, do you even notice the artwork on your walls since it's always there and you've grown accustomed to seeing it? Might changing it up, even if you move artwork to another spot in your house, make you appreciate it again since it'll be in a new space? Do you need to replace some pillows on your couch or refresh your window or shower curtains?

Taking care of your home space means taking care of your headspace.

One study found that the way people describe their homes may reflect whether their time at home feels restorative or stressful. Married women with more stressful home scores had profiles associated with adverse health outcomes. They also had increased depressed mood over the course of the day. Women with higher restorative home scores, on the other hand, had decreased depressed mood over the day.

For some, the physical act of cleaning or organizing their space releases endorphins or feel-good chemicals within the brain.

"We've evolved a preference for order and symmetry because, presumably, those things conferred an evolutionary advantage back in our ancestral environment," noted Alice Boyes, PhD, author of *The Anxiety Toolkit* and *The Healthy Mind Toolkit*, for *Psychology Today*. "When things feel out of order, it can (but not always does) make us feel scattered and anxious. Creating order relieves that anxiety."

Living with Too Much Stuff

According to Regina Lark, a professional organizer, the average U.S. household has three hundred thousand things, from paper clips to ironing boards. Let that sink in. Three hundred THOUSAND.

We can make excuses for why we need or want all these things in our home, but the reality is we likely don't. And removing things we don't need or want anymore allows us to create a space we *do* want to spend more time in. Our brains process clutter and mess as a distraction, and it holds up mental bandwidth. Removing that clutter gives your brain less to worry about and allows for more clearheaded thinking.

─────────────── TRY IT ───────────────

If your home is already clutter-free, perhaps you'll want to use this opportunity to create a space that is inviting and welcoming, brings calm to your mind and body, and encourages you to linger rather than be in a constantly hurried state.

If it's not quite as clutter-free as you'd like, consider tackling what isn't working for you first. You'd be surprised at how some small changes in your home can make a big difference.

1 CLEAR THE PHYSICAL CLUTTER TO CLEAR THE MENTAL CLUTTER. There is no shortage of books or movements to help you declutter your space. Marie Kondo, a professional organizing consultant, has sold more than four million books on the topic of tidying up our spaces. Her books, *The Life-Changing Magic of Tidying Up* and follow-up *Spark Joy*, have even rendered her last name a verb as some say they are "Kondoing" their space. Part of the appeal of her method, called the KonMari method, is it asks people to take a hard look at each and every item in their home, lay it out by category, and touch each piece before asking, "Does this item spark joy?" If you answer that it does spark joy, you can keep it. If it does not, either donate it or toss it out.

2 CARVE OUT TIME TO DECLUTTER YOUR SPACE. It does not happen overnight, but if you schedule time on your calendar to go through certain categories, you'll find yourself getting through it faster than you may have thought. For example, one category could be handbags. Just handbags. Gather any and all handbags throughout your home, and decide which to keep and which can go. Another category could be socks. Go through all your socks and decide which deserve to stay and accept which have too many holes and you'll never mend them so they can go. As you start seeing some gains from clearing out things or organizing, those endorphins kick in and motivate you to keep going.

3 BE HONEST WITH YOURSELF. Are you really ever going to wear that outfit again or find that missing sock or earring? Remember, it brought you joy at some point, and it can now bring joy to someone else. Or in the case of missing earrings or socks with holes that you meant to mend but will likely never find or repair, it's time to let them go. Release that item from your space and mind.

Once you clear out and organize things, go through each room and consider how you want to feel as you enter it. Keep in mind, you don't need to spend more money to create this type of comforting and inviting environment.

"I would start with items you already have and love looking at," Jamie Gold recommends. Gold is a wellness design consultant and the award-winning author of *Wellness by Design*.

Gold suggests looking at things that have some sort of meaning or remind you of a special place or situation. "Maybe that's the shells you brought back from the Caribbean or a throw your grandmother crocheted for you. Once you've selected your self-care inspiration pieces, you can search sites like Pinterest for ideas on how they can be used in a room. There are so many resources available online now. Don't make it complicated or expensive; that may end up adding to your stress instead of creating respite. Think about comfort and joy, the fifth facet of wellness design."

You want to create a self-care space in your home as it feels good to you. For some, this will mean less clutter. For others, it's to be more organized. Others still will want to be surrounded by the warmth of a fire during the cold months or windows wide open during the warmer months. It will mean more fragrant flowers or beautiful candles. More art that speaks to you when you see the piece. It could be a beautiful bookcase filled with books you've read or plan to read.

"The idea is to nurture your soul with elements that speak to love, joy, nature or the elements of life that inspire you," Gold told me. "That could be spirituality, family, literature, or music. Surrounding yourself with those elements gives you an intentional break from stress and routine."

Here are some things to think about:

* Start from the outside. Is the area leading to your door a place you can spruce up? Consider the outdoors and how it looks from inside your window as well. "Wind chimes, bird feeders,

and other outdoor elements can enhance the view from your space—or help create an outdoor self-care space," Gold said.

* As you enter your space, how does your entryway speak to your senses? Is it appealing to look at? Is there something you can include that provides a pleasing fragrance?

* Which room do you gravitate to as you come home after a long day and want to unwind? Bluetooth speakers are an inexpensive luxury that will allow you to play mood-shifting music throughout any room in your house. Live houseplants help circulate fresh air and add a beautiful natural element to your space. There are plants that do well in low light as well as more natural light. Visually, think about your lighting situation. We often think about what's on countertops or tables, but we don't always think about other things that affect our sight such as lighting. Can you install dimmable lights or use those controls more often?

* As you bring new items into your home, choose natural textiles or materials over synthetic. Look for textiles made with natural fibers such as wool, for example, or sustainable wood furniture. Synthetic materials can emit toxic fumes that are bad for our health.

* Add more comforting textiles. "Soft rugs, throws, pillows, and other comforting elements can help create a self-care space in your home," Gold added.

48

Capture a Memory

Svetlana Battaglin once read a quote that said photography is an instant memory. "I couldn't agree more," she said of the sentiment.

For some, taking photographs is more than just the still image it produces, whether using a smartphone, digital camera, or a point-and-shoot analog camera where you don't even know how the photo will turn out until the film is developed in a darkroom. It's about seeing the world through a different lens, which, in this case, happens to be a camera lens. It's about being observant of what's around you, seeing things in a different light, noticing things that you might otherwise miss, appreciating the artistry of a photo that means something to you, even if it doesn't mean anything to anyone else.

Battaglin recalls taking a walk along Lake Michigan with her mother and having a mother-daughter discussion when she suddenly paused because she was drawn to some cracks that formed on the sidewalk. They appeared as abstracts in her mind. She immediately pulled out the phone from her pocket, admitting that to a certain extent, she was ignoring her mom at this point. She framed the shot and took a few images to see if she was able to capture as a photo what she was seeing in front of her. Her mother was taken aback because she didn't see what was so captivating to her until Battaglin showed her the pictures.

Although she didn't take a picture of the two of them together, when Battaglin looks at these pictures, she says it reminds her of the discussion with her mother. "I captured a moment that only I will understand," Battaglin admitted. If someone else saw those images, they may trigger a completely different set of memories or not trigger anything at all. "In my opinion, that's where the power of photography lies," she told me.

Sometimes things we see right in front of us aren't as obvious until we pause to really appreciate our surroundings. Consider going for a walk when we need a break and want to get outside. We may be walking but our thinking minds don't rest. We're still trying to process something in our minds. Bringing along a camera or taking out our smartphones gives us a reason to pause and really soak in our surroundings. To observe what's in front of and around us rather than walking aimlessly.

In recent years, social media platforms like Instagram have encouraged amateur photographers to participate in a daily photo challenge in which they're invited to upload one photo a day and tag it #365 (so they can find and engage with others who are participating in the challenge). There has been some debate about whether using your smartphone to document daily images takes you away from being in the moment, but research suggests otherwise.

A study published in *Health: An Interdisciplinary Journal for the Social Study of Health, Illness and Medicine* and coauthored by Dr. Liz Brewster of Lancaster University and Dr. Andrew Cox of the University of Sheffield found that taking a photo a day and publishing it on social media improved well-being through self-care and community interaction and allowed for the potential for reminiscence. Part of the reason is you have to take a moment to take an image, and you're actively seeking something unique throughout your day to share on social media. Then once you upload it and tag it, you're able to engage with others. There is an inherent community built into the images people are sharing from around the world as you engage with others based on images they've taken as well as responding to feedback you receive on images you share.

According to one participant from the study, "My job was a very highly stressful role… There were some days when I'd almost not stopped to breathe, you know what I mean… And just the thought: oh wait a moment, no, I'll stop and take a photograph of this insect sitting on my computer or something. Just taking a moment is very salutary I think."

Another participant remarked that taking a photo a day encouraged her to get out of the house when she would be just as comfortable sitting indoors with a cup of tea. "I'll think maybe I'll take a walk down to the seafront and before I know it I'm two miles along the coast."

Just as you feel flipping through an old-school photo album and remembering times from long ago, scrolling back through the images you've taken allows you to remember the time you took each image. Seeing a photo again brings you back to how you were feeling or what you were going through at the time you took it.

One needn't rely on social media to enjoy the benefits of taking photos. "We show that, relative to not taking photos, photography can heighten enjoyment of positive experiences by increasing engagement," wrote Kristin Diehl, PhD, of the University of Southern California, Gal Zauberman, PhD, of Yale University, and Alixandra Barasch, PhD, of the University of Pennsylvania in a study published in the *Journal of Personality and Social Psychology*.

It's understandable to think pausing to take photographs would detract from the experience, but the study found that participants who took photos reported being more engaged in the activity. "One critical factor that has been shown to affect enjoyment is the extent to which people are engaged with the experience," the authors wrote. Instead of detracting from their experience, they found that taking photos naturally draws people more into the experience.

While Battaglin considers herself an amateur photographer and photography a recreational hobby, she admits that it, as well as some other hobbies, represents a creative outlet that helps her with work-life balance. She often takes photos on her walks or places she visits and admits she's very observant when she's out and about. If she sees something that captures her attention, she'll take a shot with a camera or her phone to document the object or moment. She likes to share her pictures with friends and family because it also invites engagement and discussions with them.

——————— TRY IT ———————

1. Start by taking pictures of things you're interested in, and play with the settings and composition. And be patient with yourself and your camera as you learn. Eventually, pulling out your camera will become second nature.

2. Consider taking images from different perspectives, even if they look "off" to you. You never know what you'll see until after you click the button.

3. Remember, photography is an art form, and you can be creative with your approach. There is no right or wrong angle to take a shot. Allow yourself to be inspired. Experiment, document, share to a social media platform, or don't. It's entirely up to you what you do with your photos.

4. If you miss a shot or it didn't come out the way you wanted it to, don't worry. "Keep calm, keep going, and don't give up," Battaglin said.

5. Finally, be patient with yourself and your camera. The best part is you might end up with images that bring back great memories, either for your own enjoyment or to share with others.

SEE

49

Building Community

G iving back and being part of a community that accepts you, looks forward to seeing you, and doesn't care about your history, how much money you make, or where (or if) you went to college can be incredibly powerful in supporting our health and well-being. Seeing the same parent at the school pickup line, talking with your favorite barista when you order your morning coffee, or volunteering at your place of faith and seeing familiar faces helps build our community, and that gives us a stronger sense of purpose and belonging. It allows us to not feel like strangers. Engaging with others and making real-world connections releases hormones that contribute to our mood and well-being.

In short, we need to feel part of a community. Now more than ever.

Christina Schleich understands the power of community

building and the impact it has on neighbors. As the lead organizer of the Avondale Gardening Association, a hyperlocal urban agriculture organization on Chicago's northwest side, she helps bridge those connections by organizing events throughout the year, from swapping garden seeds to inviting neighbors to care for community chickens.

Recognizing not everyone is eager to meet new people in person, Schleich offers different ways for people to get involved. Zoom events over the winter months allow people to get to know each other in a way that isn't intimidating. For larger in-person events, she'll often ask people if they want a role to play because she's found they're more comfortable in a social space if they have a defined purpose.

"We really do try to engage people where they're most comfortable so that we can more fully engage them," Schleich told me.

While it's not unique to renters, one study showed 43 percent of home renters wish they were more connected to their neighbors, while nearly 50 percent wanted to live where they could give back and feel close to their neighbors. Despite this desire, many struggle to make these connections, relying on social media to get their updates.

Those connections with others and recognizing familiar faces aren't just niceties. They can be our lifelines in times of need. Mental Health America found that 71 percent of people surveyed turned to friends or family in times of stress.

As social animals, we crave feeling supported, valued, and connected. We want to be seen.

How does one go about creating those connections in

cities like Chicago? Chicago is a big city with big-city problems. Schleich has no illusions that she can save the city from its ills. But she's got her sights on helping her own neighborhood and doing everything she can to make those connections. "I can't change Chicago, but I can change Avondale if I talk to my neighbors," she insisted. And for those who don't think that's enough, she argues that in a lot of ways, making those closer connections matters more since we have so much more impact out our front door.

Don't let our "connections" via our social media platforms fool you. We may be "connected" to more people, but those connections are no match for the time we spend with people in real life, whether it's gardening alongside our neighbors to beautify a corner lot at the end of the block or volunteering at a local food pantry.

When we see each other, when we meet up with others, we share more than common interests. We also share what's been going on in our lives, learn what's going on within our community, and feel like we're part of something bigger than ourselves. Our contributions and practicing kindness to our fellow community members are appreciated, and that makes us feel good.

Practicing kindness can jump-start several "happy" hormones, from oxytocin to dopamine and serotonin. While most people know oxytocin as the "love hormone," in this case, it plays a role in forming social bonds and trusting people, which also helps lower our blood pressure.

Dr. Waguih William IsHak, professor of psychiatry at Cedars-Sinai, notes that studies have also linked random acts of kindness to releasing dopamine, a chemical messenger in the brain that can give us a feeling of euphoria. "This feel-good brain chemical is credited with causing what's known as a 'helper's high,'" he explained. "In addition to boosting oxytocin and dopamine, being kind can also increase serotonin, a neurotransmitter that helps regulate mood."

In another report, Debra Umberson and Jennifer Karas Montez, sociology researchers at the University of Texas at Austin, noted that social relationships—both quantity and quality—affect mental health, health behavior, physical health, and mortality risk.

According to the *Harvard Women's Health Watch*, social connections like family gatherings or seeing each other in person by getting together as part of a community give us pleasure and influence our long-term health in ways every bit as powerful as adequate sleep, a good diet, and not smoking. "Dozens of studies have shown that people who have social support from family, friends, and their community are happier, have fewer health problems, and live longer," it reports.

What might be the reason for these biological and behavioral factors? According to the report, scientists found connecting with others helps relieve harmful levels of stress, which can adversely affect coronary arteries, gut function, insulin regulation, and the immune system. "Another line of research suggests that caring behaviors trigger the release of stress-reducing hormones."

Connecting with community members can be one of the easiest ways to strengthen your health and well-being since it's close to home and inexpensive, it aligns with your interests, and all that is required is (usually) showing up.

—————————————— TRY IT ——————————————

1 Consider what you enjoy doing or what you'd like to learn, and find a local group. You don't need to know how to do the activity. Learning with others can be half the fun. Want to learn to garden? Join a local gardening group. Love to cook? Offer to meet up with friends to cook meals for a food pantry. Try to find a group that meets regularly so you can get to know others over time.

2 As Schleich offers to her group, ask if there is a role you can play in your community or within a volunteer group. If there is an opportunity to check in people at an entrance, for example, you'll get to meet everyone and put a face with a name. Or if you can lead a demonstration or help support an activity, you'll have an active role to play while also getting to know people and feel like you are part of the group.

3 If you want to give back on a more consistent basis, consider volunteering at a local nonprofit. Helping others can be a satisfying way to give back while building friendships.

4 If you're still not feeling like you belong, ask questions. Many people want to help and might not know what you need from them. Asking questions shows you're interested in learning from them and want to be part of the group.

5 Once you're part of a group that meets regularly, your presence will be expected, and knowing people will be happy to see you can be a powerful motivator to keep showing up. We all like to feel appreciated, and knowing others are relying on us makes us feel wanted.

6 Give it time, and keep showing up. While some people report instant friendships formed after an initial meeting, it's not unusual for some people to need more time before they're willing to let their guard down. According to IsHak, while the simple act of kindness can reward our bodies and minds with those feel-good chemical substances, in order for them to continue, our activity needs to become a regular practice. "The rewards of acts of kindness are many," IsHak says. "They help us feel better and they help those who receive them. We're building better selves and better communities at the same time."

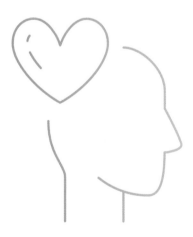

Do Nothing

The idea of doing nothing, when I have so much I need to do, seems preposterous to me. And yet I was so drawn to Olga Mecking's book, *Niksen: Embracing the Dutch Art of Doing Nothing,* for that very reason. Maybe it was because I didn't want to have so much on my plate. Maybe it was because I want the chance to do...nothing.

But what does *doing nothing* even mean?

Mecking, a writer and author based in the Netherlands, explains doing nothing is actually multisensory, and it might help if people thought about it as grounding. Grounding, she said, is "when you focus on things you can perceive with your senses."

Another way to look at doing nothing is going for a walk because you want to enjoy the outdoors, not because you need to get ten thousand steps in that day. Or resisting the urge to pull out your phone or read a book while on the train and instead just enjoying seeing the world go by. Or sitting on your couch, looking out the window, and giving yourself permission to daydream—one of Mecking's personal favorite ways to do nothing.

Mecking calls these windows of opportunities "in between things that happen." I like to think about them as the white space in our lives. Those periods we can easily fill with something, but we don't *have* to.

In fact, some say filling those white spaces is hurting us more than benefiting us. We need that downtime, that time to be bored, so our minds have time to process what's going on around us.

"Downtime is more about 'being' in the moment with spontaneous emergence of whatever activity may or may not arise rather than 'doing' a preplanned activity with a goal or preset agenda," according to a study published in *NeuroLeadership Journal*.

Similar to Mecking's definition, the authors of the *NeuroLeadership Journal* study define *downtime* as "intentionally having no intention, of consciously engaging in doing nothing specific or 'preplanned,' a process of disconnecting from intended directions and surrendering to daydreaming, letting our minds wander off in no particular direction with spontaneity and freedom."

Manoush Zomorodi, journalist, host of TED Radio Hour, and author of *Bored and Brilliant: How Spacing Out Can Unlock Your Most Productive and Creative Self*, didn't recognize how much boredom plays a role in helping us solve issues or ignite our creativity until it was nonexistent in her life. In her TED Talk in 2017, she admitted, "By doing nothing, you are actually being your most productive and creative self. It might feel weird and uncomfortable at first, but boredom truly can lead to brilliance."

Given all the benefits of doing nothing, why is it that we're not doing more of it or find it hard to do?

"People all over the world felt guilty when they tried to do nothing," Mecking told me. "And it's a very uncomfortable feeling." She cited Timothy Wilson's "shocking" study in which people preferred to give themselves electric shocks rather than sit still with nothing to do. The University of Virginia psychologist and his colleagues discovered 67 percent of men and 25 percent of women gave themselves at least one shock during their study rather than do nothing at all.

Mecking understands societal pressure to feel like we cannot waste any time. We must be productive in all areas of life. We have to be the perfect parent, employee, partner, or friend, have a tidy house, eat the proper and nutritious foods. "It's exhausting," she added. "And from that, people have this feeling that they cannot just sit down and do nothing."

And yet it's during that downtime, that time doing nothing, that our brains can rest and catch up. "In many ways, downtime permits a sorting through of many disparate elements of our mental lives, permitting a process called integration— the linkage of differentiated parts—to naturally unfold," the study in *NeuroLeadership* added.

Mecking offers several ways to practice niksen in her book, but when I asked her for just one piece of advice to help busy and stressed people get started, she said: schedule it.

This idea seems baffling to me because the whole concept is to *not* schedule more stuff on your calendar, right? She admits it's a bit of a mind trick and attributes the tip to time management expert Laura Vanderkam, whom she also interviewed in the book.

We're trying to meet people where they are, Mecking explained. We like to schedule things. We like to check off things from our to-do list. By scheduling "nothing" on your calendar, you're essentially filling in that space on your calendar so you don't add something else to it. You treat it like you would any other important thing on your calendar, such as a meeting with your boss, attending your kid's sporting event, or exercising. "Not leaving blank spaces in your agenda kind of works the same way," Mecking offered.

To reiterate the message from the *NeuroLeadership* study: intentionally have no intention.

—————————— TRY IT ——————————

1 PLAN IT. As Mecking reminds readers in her book, if we want to prioritize doing nothing as much as we prioritize getting exercise or spending time with our family, we have to plan for some downtime. "It's time to treat your niksen time as one of the most important things on Earth," she wrote. "Your mental and physical health matter, and niksen will boost both of those."

2 FIND YOUR WHITE SPACE MOMENTS. As busy as we are, we all have time throughout the day when we have a few minutes of downtime. It could be early in the morning

before everyone wakes up or maybe right after dinner when everyone is winding down. Or it could be your daily walk to get coffee or waiting to pick up your kids from school or at the checkout line at the grocery store. Go through your day, and see when you might have those pockets of time, and rather than grab your phone to distract yourself, do nothing. Give your mind that break. Resist the urge to fill it with mindless doom scrolling or to get "one more thing done" so you can check it off your to-do list.

③ PRACTICE DAYDREAMING. Many of us have forgotten how to daydream. What came effortlessly when we were younger seems to be a challenge now. If you sit still and it feels unnatural to you, give it some time. Practice daydreaming. Look outside your window, and follow the birds. If you're walking, listen to the sounds around you. Take some time and see where your mind takes you.

④ GIVE IT FIVE MINUTES. If it truly is hard to find a pocket of thirty minutes to do nothing, don't despair. Try five minutes. Try ten minutes. Or try splitting your time with a morning session and an afternoon session. The more often you do it, the greater the benefit.

⑤ TRY AGAIN TOMORROW. And if it just didn't happen today, try again tomorrow. Keep scheduling it on your calendar, and like any other habit you form that helps calm your body and mind, you'll start to realize doing nothing is an important part of your health and wellness tool kit.

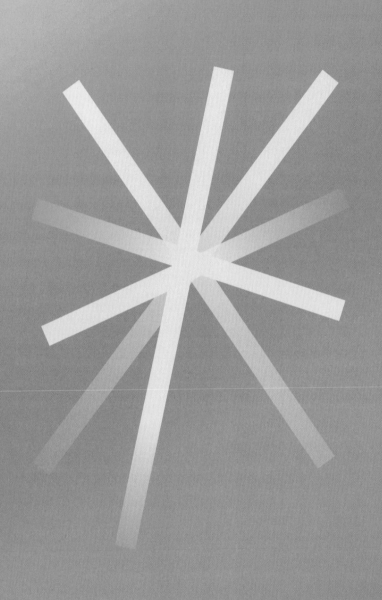

ACKNOWLEDGMENTS

True happiness isn't about being happy all the time and stress isn't always bad. Finding joy and a deeper purpose can be more fulfilling and contribute to greater happiness and well-being. Surrounding yourself with people who love and support and believe in you goes a long way, and I'm so lucky to have struck gold in that part of my life.

I can't thank my book editor, Erin McClary, enough for believing and supporting this book from the beginning and helping bring it to life, or my literary agent, Marilyn Allen, who shepherded the entire process. Immense gratitude to my Alpha Bitches, my writing ride-or-die pals who celebrated my highs and consoled me during my lows including Debbie Carlson, Kelly James, Cindy Kuzma, Aimee Levitt, Dawn Reiss, Hilary Shenfeld, Kate Silver, Jamie Sotonoff Bartosch, and Claire Zulkey. Other writer friends who inspired me to keep going and supported me in various ways include David Hochman, whose UPOD Academy changed the trajectory of my writing career, and my UPOD goats, especially Laura Shin and Vanessa McGrady. My active involvement with the American Society of Journalists and Authors has allowed me to connect with so many talented writers and editors and my PR friends, Shannan Hofman Bunting, Orly Telisman, Robin Monsky, and Jeff Salzgeber, who've been hearing me talk about this book every time we get together. Much thanks to my therapist, Danielle Burks, whose wisdom and support does not go unnoticed.

Thank you to my kids, Chloe and Alex, who listened patiently (as patiently as teenagers can) as I shared updates and sometimes dragged them with me to try many of the tips included in this book. To my parents, Helen and Chriss, and brother, Harry, who believed in me from the very beginning. Finally, this book would not have been possible without the endless support (and conversations fueled with coffee and long walks) of my husband and partner in life, Matthew Krecun. Thank you for always being my first reader, my confidante, and willing to try all my quirky ideas. Who knew some of them would end up in a book?

NOTES

INTRODUCTION

In a series: Fariss Samarrai, "Doing Something Is Better Than Nothing for Most People, Study Shows," *UVA Today*, July 3, 2014, https://news.virginia.edu /content/doing-something-better-doing -nothing-most-people-study-shows.

"The mind is designed": Samarrai, "Doing Something Is Better Than Nothing."

TOUCH

"If you truly": Sherra Aguirre *Joyful, Delicious, Vegan: Life without heart disease* (Berkeley: She Writes Press, 2021), 45.

"When you're in the garden": Ron Finley, "Meet Your Instructor," MasterClass , accessed May 21, 2023, https://www.masterclass.com/classes /ron-finley-teaches-gardening/chapters/meet-your-instructor-b50c7011-d9ec -42b5-bcdf-75f8cf309430.

According to Minneapolis-based firm Axiom: "2021 Gardening Insights Survey: Gardening in a COVID-19 World," Axiom Marketing, accessed May 21, 2023, https://axiomcom.com/2021-garden-survey/

Axiom Marketing's research: Linel Reiber, "2022 Axiom Marketing Insights Research:GrowingMorein2022,"AxiomMarketing,October11,2022,https:// axiomcom.com/axiom-gardening-insights-survey-growing-more-in-2022/.

"Engagement with both wild": Carly J. Wood, Jules Pretty, and Murray Griffin, "A Case-Control Study of the Health and Wellbeing Benefits of Allotment Gardening," *Journal of Public Health* 38, no. 3 (September 17, 2016): e336– e344, https://doi.org/10.1093/pubmed/fdv146.

While working: C. A. Lowry et al., "Identification of an Immune-Responsive Mesolimbocortical Serotonergic System: Potential Role in Regulation of Emotional Behavior," *Neuroscience* 146, no. 2 (2007): 756–72, https://doi .org/10.1016/j.neuroscience.2007.01.067.

"While we know": Shawna Coronado, *The Wellness Garden: Grow, Eat, and Walk Your Way to Better Health* (Minneapolis: Cool Springs Press, 2017), 121.

Some of those positive effects: James W. Pennebaker (social psychologist, University of Texas at Austin), in discussion with the author, December 2021.

"These improvements": Siri Carpenter, "A New Reason for Keeping A Diary," *Monitor on Psychology* 32, no. 8 (September 2001): 68, https://www.apa.org /monitor/sep01/keepdiary.

The study's results: Carpenter, "A New Reason."

"One important sign": Pennebaker.

"You are writing for yourself": Pennebaker.

Anything can be a topic: Julia Cameron, *The Right to Write* (New York: Penguin, 1998).

Yet research shows: Jackie Andrade, "What Does Doodling Do?," *Applied Cognitive Psychology* 24, no. 1 (2010): 100–06, https://doi.org/10.1002/acp .1561.

Then, Clarke wrote: David Greenberg, *Presidential Doodles: Two Centuries of Scribbles, Scratches, Squiggles and Scrawls from the Oval Office* (New York: Basic Books, 2007), 12.

Hambrick admits: Liz Hambrick (artist), in discussion with the author, January 14, 2022.

Depression, however: Hambrick.

"The experience is": Dana DuMont (artist and educator), in discussion with the author, January 15, 2022.

Engaging in mindfulness: Daphne M. Davis and Jeffrey A. Hayes, "What Are the Benefits of Mindfulness? A Practice Review of Psychotherapy-Related Research," *Psychotherapy* 48, no. 2 (2011): 198–20, https://doi.org/10.1037 /a0022062.

"I feel free": Michele Weldon (journalist and author), in discussion with the author, January 14, 2022.

In 2009: Rick J. Scheidt, "I Remember Better When I Paint," *Gerontologist* 56, no. 5 (October 2016): 968–69, https://doi.org/10.1093/geront/gnw122.

"When they are given paints": Scheidt, "I Remember Better When I Paint."

"Like mindfulness": Lydia G. Fogo, "Engagement with the Visual Arts Increases Mindfulness" (honors thesis, University of Tennessee at Chattanooga, 2017), 23, https://scholar.utc.edu/honors-theses/106/.

One study noted: Neville Owen et al., "Too Much Sitting: The Population Health Science of Sedentary Behavior," *Exercise and Sport Sciences Reviews* 38, no. 3 (July 2010): 105–13, https://doi.org/10.1097/JES.0b013e3181e373a2.

Perhaps surprising: Owen et al., "Too Much Sitting."

Movement, including dance: Erica Hornthal (dance/movement therapist and clinical professional counselor), in discussion with the author, February 8, 2022.

"It dampens that cortisol": Melissa Blount, PhD (clinical psychologist), in discussion with the author, January 14, 2022.

"I hated everything": Shannon Downey (artist, activist, founder of Badass Cross Stitch), in discussion with the author, December 14, 2021.

"One study published": D. R. Major, "On the Affective Tone of Simple Sense-Impressions," *The American Journal of Psychology* 7, no. 1 (October 1895): 57-77, https://www.jstor.org/stable/1412037.

Downey isn't alone: Jill Riley, Betsan Corkhill, and Clare Morris, "The Benefits of Knitting for Personal and Social Wellbeing in Adulthood: Findings from an International Survey," *British Journal of Occupational Therapy* 76, no. 2 (February 2013): 50–57, https://doi.org/10.4276/0308022 13X13603244419077.

"It is based": Mark Smithivas (entrepreneur), in discussion with the author, January 17, 2022.

"I get into": Dr. David Berv (chiropractic sports physician), in discussion with the author, January 17, 2022.

"Floatation-REST": Justin S. Feinstein et al., "Examining the Short Term Anxiolytic and Antidepressant Effect of Floatation-REST," *PLOS ONE* 13, no. 2 (February 2018): e0190292, https://doi.org/10.1371/journal. pone.0190292.

While the research: Mandy Oaklander, "Float Hopes: The Strange New Science of Floating," *Time*, 2015, https://time.com/floating/.

According to some research: George A. Eby III and Karen L. Eby, "Magnesium for Treatment Resistant Depression: A Review .and Hypothesis," *Medical Hypotheses* 74, no. 4 (April 2010: 649–60, https://doi.org/10.1016/j.mehy .2009.10.051.

Rhonda Mattox, MD: Elizabeth Yuko, "4 Beneficial Uses for Epsom Salt—and One You Should Always Avoid," *Real Simple*, updated October 19, 2022, https://www.realsimple.com/health/preventative-health/aches-pains/health -benefits-of-epsom-salts.

According to Feinstein's research: Feinstein et al., "Examining the Short-Term."

"She knows my body": KJ Hardy (therapist), in discussion with the author, January 9, 2022.

Aside from the benefits: Smithivas.

One study: Tiffany Field et al., "Cortisol Decreases and Serotonin and Dopamine Increase Following Massage Therapy," *International Journal of Neuroscience* 115, no. 10 (July 2009): 1397–1413, https://doi.org/ 10.1080 /00207450590956459.

According to the Mayo Clinic: "Massage Therapy," Mayo Clinic, March 3, 2023, https://www.mayoclinic.org/healthy-lifestyle/stress-management/in-depth /massage/art -20045743.

For example: Karen J. Sherman et al., "Five-Week Outcomes from a Dosing Trial of Therapeutic Massage for Chronic Neck Pain," *Annals of Family Medicine* 12, no. 2 (March 2014): 112–20, https://doi.org/10.1370/afm.1602.

Another study: Maria Meier et al., "Standardized Massage Interventions as Protocols for the Induction of Psychophysiological Relaxation in the

Laboratory: A Block Randomized, Controlled Trial," *Scientific Reports* 10, (2020): 14774, https://doi.org/10.1038/s41598-020-71173-w.

It's not uncommon: Gail Adduci Gogliotti (clinical counselor and dance/movement therapist), in discussion with the author, April 6, 2022.

"It's like having a project": Jenifer Knox (professional organizer), in discussion with the author, April 14, 2022.

The study found: "Chore or Stress Reliever: Study Suggests that Washing Dishes Decreases Stress," *Florida State University News*, September 30, 2015, https://news.fsu.edu/news/health-medicine /2015/09/30/chore-stress-reliever-study -suggests-washing-dishes -decreases-stress/.

In her piece: Ellen Byron, "Sick of Cleaning? Turn It into Meditation," *Wall Street Journal*, May 27, 2020, https://www.wsj.com/articles/sick -of-cleaning-turn-it-into-meditation-11590571801.

Until then: Ashley Fetters, "The Problem with This Year's Most Comfortable Holiday Fad," *The Atlantic*, December 17, 2018, https://www.theatlantic.com /health/archive/2018/12/weighted-blanket-history-holiday-gift/578347/.

"The chute provided": "Temple Grandin Hug Machine: How Did Weighted Blanket Research Begin?", TruHugs Shop, December 19, 2020, https://truhugs.com/research-science/do-weighted-blankets-work-temple-grandin -hugging-machine/.

In Grandin's report: Temple Grandin, "Calming Effects of Deep Touch Pressure in Patients with Autistic Disorder, College Students, and Animals," *Journal of Child and Adolescent Psychopharmacology* 2, no. 1 (January 1992): 63–72, https://doi.org/10.1089/cap.1992.2.63.

"Pressure is calming": "#AskTemple: A Live Google Hangout with CSU's Temple Grandin," Colorado State University, streamed live on April 13, 2015, YouTube video, 56:49, https://www.youtube.com/watch?v=3xHluhQ jcaQ&t=0s.

"The pressure": Dalvin Brown, "Weighted Blankets: Here's How the Trendy Bedding Got So Popular," *USA Today*, January 26, 2019, https://www .usatoday.com/story/news/nation/2019/01/26/weighted-blankets-makers -weigh-products-sudden-success /2558957002/.

According to its Kickstarter campaign: "Gravity: The Weighted Blanket for Sleep, Stress and Anxiety," Kickstarter, July 8, 2020, https://www.kickstarter.com /projects/1620645203/gravity-the-weighted-blanket-for-sleep-stress-and /posts.

Time magazine: Jamie Ducharme, "Best Inventions 2018: Blankets That Ease Anxiety: Gravity Blanket," *Time*, accessed March 24, 2022, https://time.com /collection/best-inventions-2018/5454469/gravity-blanket/.

Weighted blankets: Rahul Rao, "What the Science Actually Says about Weighted Blankets," *Popular Science*, January 26, 2021, https://www.popsci.com/story /science/weighted-blankets -anxiety/.

One study found: Annette L. Becklund, Lisa Rapp-McCall, and Jessica Nudo, "Using Weighted Blankets in an Inpatient Mental Health Hospital to Decrease

Anxiety," *Journal of Integrative Medicine* 19, no. 2 (2021): 129–34, https://doi
.org/10.1016/j.joim.2020.11.004.

"This study found": Becklund, Rapp-McCall, and Nudo, "Using Weighted Blankets."

"The pressure of": "4 Ways Weighted Blankets Can Actually Help You," *Penn Medicine,* March 24, 2022, https://www.pennmedicine.org/updates/blogs /health-and-wellness/2019/february/weighted-blankets.

"I watched people": Rao, "What the Science Actually Says."

One study showed: Brian Mullen et al., "Exploring the Safety and Therapeutic Effects of Deep Pressure Stimulation Using a Weighted Blanket," *Occupational Therapy in Mental Health* 24, no. 1 (September 2008), 65–89, https://doi .org/10.1300/J004v24 n01_05.

"We are always exploring": Emily Vincent, "Writing Power: Kent State Professor Studies Benefits of Writing Gratitude Letters," Kent State University, 2014, http://einside.kent.edu/Management%20Update%20Archive/news /announcements/success/toepferwriting.html.

Results from the research: Steven Toepfer, Kelly Cichy, and Patti Peters, "Letters of Gratitude: Further Evidence for Author Benefits," *Journal of Happiness Studies* 13, no. 1 (2012): 187–201, https://psycnet.apa.org/doi/10.1007/s10902-011 -9257-7.

By writing these letters: Vincent, "Writing Power."

So instead of taking: Amit Kumar and Nicholas Epley, "Undervaluing Gratitude: Expressers Misunderstand the Consequences of Showing Appreciation," *Psychological Science* 29, no. 9 (September 2018): 1423–35, https://doi .org/10.1177/09567 97618772506.

"Expressing gratitude": Kumar and Epley, "Undervaluing Gratitude."

Rogers and his friends: "LetsGoBtown," Correspondence Club of Bloomington, July 3, 2016, YouTube video, 4:58, https://www.youtube.com/watch?v=pp B1KoXh7ug.

"Cats are very much": Jim Horst (cat enthusiast and pet shelter volunteer), in discussion with the author, May 20, 2022.

Research has shown: Patricia Pendry and Jaymie L. Vandagriff, "Animal Visitation Program (AVP) Reduces Cortisol Levels of University Students: A Randomized Controlled Trial." *AERA Open* 5, no. 2 (June 2019), https://doi .org/10.1177/2332858419852592.

Additional insights shared: "The Friend Who Keeps You Young," John Hopkins Medicine, 2022, https://www.hopkinsmedicine.org/health/wellness-and -prevention/the-friend-who-keeps -you-young.

"The cortisol-lowering": "The Friend Who Keeps You Young."

NIH News in Health: "The Power of Pets: Health Benefits of Human-Animal Interactions," *NIH News in Health,* February 2018, https://newsinhealth.nih .gov/2018/02/power-pets.

"There's not one answer": "The Power of Pets."

"Puzzles and games": Douglas Scharre, "How Games Like Wordle Can Improve Brain Health," Ohio State University, February 9, 2022, https://health.osu.edu/health/brain-and-spine/how-games-like-wordle-can-improve-brain-health.

The "use it or lose it": Scharre, "How Games like Wordle."

"In their small": Scharre, "How Games like Wordle."

She visited the store: Blount , discussion.

"Jigsaw puzzling": Patrick Fissler et al., "Jigsaw Puzzling Taps Multiple Cognitive Abilities and Is a Potential Protective Factor for Cognitive Aging," *Frontiers of Aging Neuroscience* 10, (October 2018): 299, https://doi.org/10.3389/fnagi.2018.00299.

"The friendly": Shannan Hofman Bunting (board game enthusiast), in discussion with the author, April 18, 2022.

According to the manufacturer: "Ticket to Ride," Days of Wonder, accessed May 16, 2022, https://www.daysofwonder.com/tickettoride/en/usa/.

"I liken the art": Lesa Dowd (book binder and conservator), in discussion with the author, September 16, 2022.

"Bookbinding is an excellent craft": William Rush Dunton Jr., *Occupation Therapy: A Manual for Nurses* (Philadelphia: W. B. Saunders, 1918), 156.

With titles like: Bitter Lemon Bindery, https://www.youtube.com/c/bittermelonbindery.

"Yoga goes beyond": DuShaun Branch (founder of Sage Gawd Collective), in discussion with the author, April 18, 2022.

"When you're dealing with": Amy Guth (journalist/screenwriter/producer), in discussion with the author, May 4, 2022.

"Yoga means to yoke.": Lisa Faremouth Weber (yoga therapist), in discussion with the author, April 14, 2022.

One study reported: Clare Collins, "Yoga: Intuition, Preventive Medicine, and Treatment," *Journal of Obstetric, Gynecological & Neonatal Nursing* 27, no. 5 (September–October 1998): 563–68, https://doi.org/10.1111/j.1552-6909.1998.tb02623.x.

Results from another study: Catherine Woodyard, "Exploring the Therapeutic Effects of Yoga and Its Ability to Increase Quality of Life," *International Journal of Yoga* 4, no. 2 (2011): 49–54, https://doi.org/10.4103/0973-6131.85485.

"Tinker means playing": Alan Castel, "Tinkering Can Lead to Creative Insight and Innovation," *Psychology Today*, April 23, 2020, https://www.psychologytoday.com/us/blog/metacognition-and-the-mind/202004/tinkering-can-lead-creative-insight-and -innovation.

"For me": Brian Carberry (editor), in discussion with the author, January 7, 2022.

"In life": Castel, "Tinkering."

"I started to sand it": Vanessa McGrady (writer), in discussion with the author, May 23, 2022.

Even if solutions: Simone M. Ritter and Ap Dijksterhuis, "Creativity—The Unconscious Foundations of the Incubation Period," *Frontiers in*

Human Neuroscience 8, (April 2014): 215, https://doi.org/10.3389/fnhum .2014.00215.

"Mind wandering": Castel, "Tinkering."

When he ran track: Ken Monarrez (runner), in discussion with the author, May 26, 2022.

"Most of the time": Cindy Kuzma (runner, journalist, podcaster, and author), in discussion with the author, May 22, 2022.

Among the experts: Scott Douglas, *Running Is My Therapy: Relieve Stress and Anxiety, Fight Depression, Ditch Bad Habits and Live Happier* (New York: The Experiment, 2018), 60.

Ekkekakis also notes: Douglas, *Running Is My Therapy*, 82

People often talk: Douglas, *Running Is My Therapy*, 84.

TASTE

Moonlynn Tsai: Carolyn L. Todd and Esther Tseng, "Eat Well: 16 People Redefining Healthy Eating," *Self,* March 30, 2021, https://www.self.com /story/eat-well.

Mahatma Ghandi once said: Maryn Liles, "125 Inspiring Mahatma Ghandi Quotes That'll Change Your Life," *Parade,* October 31, 2022, https://parade. com/1247073/marynliles/gandhi-quotes.

"Slow food brings together": Anna Mulé (executive director of Slow Food USA), in discussion with the author, February 22, 2022.

According to one study: Jessica Martino, Jennifer Pegg, and Elizabeth Pegg Frates, "The Connection Prescription: Using the Power of Social Interactions and the Deep Desire for Connectedness to Empower Health and Wellness," *American Journal of Lifestyle Medicine* 11, no. 6 (October 2015): 466–75, https://doi.org/10.1177/1559827615608788.

"Lingering and connecting": Brekke Bounds (board member of Slow Food Chicago), in discussion with the author, February 16, 2022.

Quince, dates: C. Prasad, "Food, Mood and Health: A Neurobiological Outlook," *Brazilian Journal of Medical and Biological Research* 31, no. 12 (1998): 1517–27, https://pubmed.ncbi.nlm.nih.gov/9951546/.

In turn: Sarah-Marie Hopf, "You Are What You Eat: How Food Affects Your Mood," *Dartmouth Undergraduate Journal of Science,* February 3, 2011, https:// sites.dartmouth.edu/dujs/2011/02/03/you-are-what-you-eat-how-food -affects-your-mood./

"Serotonin is an important": Hopf, "You Are What You Eat."

"Chocolate contains": Carol Ottley, "Food and Mood," *Nursing Standard* 15, no. 2 November (2000): 46–52, http://doi.org/10.7748/ldp2000.11.3.4.32. c1438.

What's likely at play: M. Macht and D. Dettmer, "Everyday Mood and Emotions after Eating a Chocolate Bar or an Apple," *Appetite* 46, no. 3 May May (2006): 332–36, https://doi.org/10.1016/j.appet.2006.01.014.

Caffeine, on the other hand: Jenna Fletcher, "What to Know about the Different

Types of Psychoactive Drugs," *Medical News Today*, May 19, 2022, https://www.medicalnewstoday.com/articles/types-of-psychoactive-drugs.

Roughly 80 percent: "Caffeine and Long Work Hours," Centers for Disease Control and Prevention, April 1, 2020, https://www.cdc.gov/niosh/emres/longhourstraining/caffeine.html.

For many of us: Fletcher, "What to Know."

While it can calm: Fletcher, "What to Know."

There is a reason: P. J. Rogers and H. M. Lloyd, "Nutrition and Mental Performance," *Proceedings of the Nutrition Society* 53, no. 2 (July 1994): 443–56, https://doi.org/10.1079/pns19940049.

In one study: C. Michaud et al., "Effects of Breakfast Size on Short-Term Memory Concentration and Blood Glucose," *Journal of Adolescent Health* 12, no. 1 (January 1991): 53–57, https://doi.org/10.1016/0197-0070(91)90042-k.

"Think of the last time": Heather L. Nickrand (hospice regional bereavement and volunteer manager with AMITA Health), in discussion with the author, December 1, 2021.

Cooking and baking: Jeanne Whalen, "A Road to Mental Health through the Kitchen," *Wall Street Journal*, December 8, 2014, https://www.wsj.com/articles/a-road-to-mental-health-through -the-kitchen-1418059204.

In a study published: Ann Futterman Collier and Heidi A. Wayment, "Psychological Benefits of the 'Maker' or Do-It-Yourself Movement in Young Adults: A Pathway Towards Subjective Well-Being," *Journal of Happiness Studies* 19, (April 2018): 1217–39, https://doi.org/10.1007/s10902-017-9866-x.

"Preparing a meal": Linda Wasmer Andrews, "Kitchen Therapy: Cooking Up Mental Well-Being," *Psychology Today*, May 19, 2015, https://www.psychologytoday.com/us/blog/minding-the-body/201505/kitchen-therapy -cooking- mental-well-being.

"You weigh out": Jennifer Billock (author of *Historic Chicago Bakeries*), in discussion with the author, May 19, 2022.

While research continues: Yong-Hyun Ko et al., "Flavonoids as Therapeutic Candidates for Emotional Disorders such as Anxiety and Depression," *Archives of Pharmacal Research* 43, no. 11 (November 2020): 1128–43, https://doi.org/10.1007/s12272-020-01292-5.

Some studies show: Shinsuke Hidese et al., "Effects of L-Theanine Administration on Stress-Related Symptoms and Cognitive Functions in Healthy Adults: A Randomized Controlled Trial," *Nutrients* 11, no. 10 (October 2019): 2362, https://doi.org/10.3390/nu11102362.

Daily cups: Andrew Steptoe et al., "The Effects of Tea on Psychophysiological Stress Responsivity and Post-Stress Recovery: A Randomised Double-Blind Trial," *Psychopharmacology* 190, (2007): 81–89, https://doi.org/10.1007/s00213-006-0573-2.

The study suggests: "Black Tea Soothes Away Stress," UCL News, October 4, 2006, https://www.ucl.ac.uk/news/2006/oct/black-tea-soothes-away-stress.

"In large doses": Lisa Wartenberg, "How Much Caffeine Does Tea Have Compared with Coffee?," *Healthline,* October 7, 2019, https://www.health line.com/nutrition/caffeine-in-tea-vs-coffee.

"and migraines": Ann I. Scher, Walter F. Stewart, and Richard B. Lipton, "Caffeine as a Risk Factor for Chronic Daily Headache: A Population-Based Study," *Neurology* 63, no. 11 (December 2004): 2022–27, https://doi .org/10.1212/01.wnl.0000145760.37852.ed.

"To my mind": Kaumudi Marathé (chef/writer), in discussion with the author, April 28, 2022.

According to one study: T. Alan Jiang, "Health Benefits of Culinary Herbs and Spices," *Journal of AOAC International* 102, no. 2 (March 2019): 395–411, https://doi.org/10.5740/jaoacint.18 -0418.

As the study reported: Jiang, "Health Benefits."

It might have been: Mark Lucock, "Is Folic Acid the Ultimate Functional Food Component for Disease Prevention?" *BMJ* 328, no. 7433 (January 24, 2004): 211-4, https://doi.org/10.1136/bmj.328.7433.211.

Dr. Eva Selhub: Eva Selhub, "Nutritional Psychiatry: Your Brain on Food," Harvard Health Publishing, March 26, 2020, https://www.health.harvard. edu/blog/nutritional-psychiatry-your-brain-on-food-201511168626.

"Diets high in": Selhub, "Nutritional Psychiatry."

The "gut-brain axis": Sean Rossman, "These Foods Will Boost Your Mood and Make You Happy," *USA Today,* May 9, 2017, https://www.usatoday.com /story/news/nation-now/2017/05/09/foods-make-you-happy/307583001/.

"We're realizing": Rossman, "These Foods."

By making sure: Selhub, "Nutritional Psychiatry."

How do we do this?: Gina Caruso (integrative nutrition health coach), in discussion with the author, March 16, 2022.

Many of these unprocessed foods: Selhub, "Nutritional Psychiatry."

A meta-analysis: Jun S. Lai et al., "A Systematic Review and Meta Analysis of Dietary Patterns and Depression in Community-Dwelling Adults," *American Journal of Clinical Nutrition* 99, no. 1 (January 2014): 181–97, https://doi .org/10.3945/ajcn .113.069880.

Another study found: Felice N. Jacka et al., "A Randomised Controlled Trial of Dietary Improvement for Adults with Major Depression (the 'SMILES' Trial)," *BMC Medicine* 15, (January 2017): 23, https://doi.org/10.1186/s12916-017-0791-y.

The *World Journal of Psychiatry* published: Laura R. LaChance and Drew Ramsey, "Antidepressant Foods: An Evidence-Based Nutrient Profiling System for Depression," *World Journal of Psychiatry* 8, no. 3 (September 2018): 97–104, https://doi.org/10.5498/wjp .v8.i3.97.

According to Epel: Jill Suttie, "Better Eating through Mindfulness," *Greater Good Magazine,* June 27, 2012, https://greatergood.berkeley.edu/article /item/better_eating_through_mind fulness.

"Stress affects": Suttie, "Better Eating through Mindfulness."

"Feeling stressed out": Susan Albers, *Eating Mindfully* (New York: MJF Books, 2012).

In another book: Susan Albers, *Eat, Drink, and Be Mindful* (New York: New Harbinger, 2008).

SMELL

If only there could be: Nina Auerbach, *Daphne du Maurier, Haunted Heiress* (Philadelphia: University of Pennsylvania Press, 1999), 64.

"It is scientifically proven": Kendall Cornish, "The Benefits of Scented Candles According to a Psychotherapist," *Travel + Leisure*, May 16, 2020, https://www.travelandleisure.com/style/shopping/benefits-of-candles.

Chalkia understands: Chryssa Chalkia, "Scented Candles to Reduce Anxiety," Counselling Directory, August 28, 2018, https://www.counselling-directory.org.uk/memberarticles/scented-candles-to-reduce-anxiety.

According to *Yoga International* magazine: Natalya Podgorny, "Candlelight Insight: Trataka," *Yoga International*, 2022, https://yogainternational.com/article/view/candlelight-insight-trataka.

"Whether you lust": "About", Pine & Burn Candle Co., accessed November 18, 2022, https://www.pineandburn.com/about.

"There's sort of an inherent ritual": Amanda Glazebrook (founder of Pine and Burn Candle Company), in discussion with the author, April 5, 2022.

"The soothing effect": Chalkia, "Scented Candles."

When seeking out candles: Chalkia, "Scented Candles."

"Who didn't have a sandwich": Billock, discussion.

Ellen King understands: Ellen King (baker and author), in discussion with the author, May 24, 2022.

A report from the study: Real Bread Campaign, "Together We Rise: Bethlem Baking Buddies," Sustain, November 14, 2017, https://www.sustainweb.org/publications/togetherwerise/.

One of the reasons: Sarah Horowitz-Thran (perfumer), in discussion with the author, April 27, 2022.

"We are reassured by aromas": Sarah McCartney (perfumer and author), in discussion with the author, April 27, 2022.

And while most of us: J. Lehrner et al., "Ambient Odor of Orange in a Dental Office Reduces Anxiety and Improves Mood in Female Patients," *Physiology & Behavior* 71, no. 1–2 (October 2000): 83–86, https://doi.org/10.1016/S0031-9384(00)00308-5.

In the book McCartney cowrote: Sarah McCartney and Samantha Scriven, *The Perfume Companion: The Definitive Guide to Choosing Your Next Scent* (London: Frances Lincoln, 2021).

While essential oils: "Our History: 1880 to 1918," Gattefossé, accessed May 21, 2023, https://www.gattefosse.com/corporate-content/gattefosse-history-1880-to-1918.

Essential oils are: "Aromatherapy: Do Essential Oils Really Work?," Johns Hopkins Health, accessed January 5, 2022, https://www.hopkinsmedicine.org/health/wellness-and-prevention/aromatherapy-do-essential-oils-really-work.

"When inhaled": "Aromatherapy."

One study measured: Margaret Louis and Susan D. Kowalski, "Use of Aromatherapy with Hospice Patients to Decrease Pain, Anxiety, and Depression and to Promote an Increased Sense of Well-Being," *American Journal of Hospice and Palliative Medicine* 9, no. 6 (November 2002): 381–86, https://doi.org/10.1177/104990910201900607.

"The ability of essential oils": Lorena R. Lizarraga-Valderrama, "Effects of Essential Oils on Central Nervous System: Focus on Mental Health," *Phytotherapy Research* 35, no. 2 (2021): 657–79, https://doi.org/10.1002/ptr.6854.

Another study: Isabel Sánchez-Vidaña et al., "The Effectiveness of Aromatherapy for Depressive Symptoms: A Systematic Review," *Evidence-Based Complementary and Alternative Medicine* 2017, (2017): 5869315, https://doi.org/10.1155/2017/5869315.

Research published: Hiroki Harada et al., "Linalool Odor-Induced Anxiolytic Effects in Mice," *Frontiers in Behavioral Neuroscience* 12, (October 2018): 241, https://doi.org/10.3389/fnbeh.2018.00241.

The biggest misconception: "An Interview with Aromatherapy Experts," Taking Charge of Your Survivorship, 2022, https://www.takingcharge.csh.umn.edu/survivorship/interview-aromatherapy-experts.

The FDA classifies: "Aromatherapy," U.S. Food and Drug Administration, updated February 25, 2022, https://www.fda.gov/cosmetics/cosmetic-products/aromatherapy.

Start with very small: "Interview with Aromatherapy Experts."

"Nature therapy": Brenda Spitzer (forest therapy guide), in discussion with the author, October 29, 2021.

Some researchers found: Marc G. Berman, John Jonides, and Stephen Kaplan, "The Cognitive Benefits of Interacting with Nature," *Psychological Science* 19, no. 12 (December 2008):1207, https://doi.org/10.1111/j.1467-9280.2008.02225.x.

while other researchers: Stephen Kaplan and Marc G. Berman, "Directed Attention as a Common Resource for Executive Functioning and Self-Regulation," *Perspectives on Psychological Science* 5, no. 1 (May 2017): 43–57, https://doi.org/10.1177/1745691609356784.

According to the study: Phoebe R. Bentley et al., "Nature, Smells and Human Wellbeing," *Ambio* 52, (2023): 1–14, https://doi.org/10.1007/s13280-022-01760-w.

Conversely, living in places: J. Maas et al., "Morbidity Is Related to a Green Living Environment," *Journal of Epidemiology & Community Health* 63, no. 12 (December 2009): 96773, https://doi.org/10.1136/jech.2008.079038.

Instead of viewing: M. Amos Clifford (founder of the Association of Nature and

Forest Therapy Guides and Programs and author), in discussion with the author, November 4, 2021.

"Today, people who work": Richard Louv (author) in discussion with the author, November 28, 2021.

"The incredible thing": Joyce Shulman (walk leader and author), in discussion with the author, January 17, 2022.

Research has shown: "Walking Can Help Relieve Stress," North Dakota State University, August 8, 2011, https://www.ag.ndsu.edu/news/news releases/2011/aug-8-2011/walking-can-help -relieve-stress.

Even a short bout: Meghan K. Edwards and Paul D. Loprinzi, "Experimental Effects of Brief, Single Bouts of Walking and Meditation on Mood Profile in Young Adults," *Health Promotion Perspectives* 8, no. 3 (July 2018): 171–78, https://doi.org/10.15171/hpp.2018.23.

In her book: Annabel Streets, *52 Ways to Walk* (New York: G. P. Putnam's Sons, 2022), 47.

Walking as a regular practice: Karmel W. Choi et al., "Assessment of Bidirectional Relationships Between Physical Activity and Depression Among Adults: A 2-Sample Mendelian Randomization Study," *JAMA Psychiatry* 76, no. 4 (April 2019): 399–408, https://doi.org/10.1001/jamapsychiatry.2018.4175.

"We saw a 26% decrease": "More Evidence That Exercise Can Boost Mood," Harvard Health Publishing, May 1, 2019, https://www.health.harvard.edu /mind-and-mood/more-evidence-that-exercise-can-boost-mood.

"Flowers are, unquestionably": Jan Johnsen, *Floratopia: 110 Flower Garden Ideas for Your Yard, Patio, or Balcony* (New York: Countryman Press, 2021).

Unlike other senses: Bentley et al., "Nature, Smells, and Human Wellbeing."

"An average person": Jan Johnsen, *Gardentopia: Design Basics for Creating Beautiful Outdoor Spaces* (New York: Countryman Press, 2019).

"Wake up, connect": Maria Failla (author and podcast host), in discussion with the author, September 14, 2022.

There are several houseplants: Maria Failla, *Growing Joy: The Plant Lover's Guide to Cultivating Happiness (and Plants)* (New York: St. Martin's Essentials, 2022).

"Flowers should play": Johnsen, *Floratopia*.

If you have outdoor space: Johnsen, *Gardentopia*.

HEAR

"Silence is of different": Kristen Pond, "The Ethics of Silence in Charlotte Brontë's *Villette*," *Studies in English Literature, 1500-1900* 57, no. 4 (Autumn 2017): 771-797, https://www.jstor.org/stable/26541941.

There is no shortage: Albert Arias et al., "Systematic Review of the Efficacy of Meditation Techniques as Treatments for Medical Illness," *Journal of Alternative and Complementary Medicine* 12, no. 8 (2006): 817–32, https:// doi.org/10.1089/acm.2006.12.817.

Turns out the problem: Timothy D. Wilson et al., "Just Think: The Challenges of the Disengaged Mind," *Science* 345, no. 6192 (July 2014): 75–77, https://doi.org/10.1126/science.1250830.

"The mind is designed": Samarrai, "Doing Something Is Better than Doing Nothing."

Meditation is an umbrella term: "Meditation: A Simple, Fast Way to Reduce Stress," Mayo Clinic, April 29, 2022, https://www.mayoclinic.org/tests -procedures/meditation/in-depth/meditation/art-20045858.

Try repeating a mantra: Mandisa Jones (clinical social worker), in discussion with the author, March 17, 2022.

Research shows: Myriam V. Thoma et al., "The Effect of Music on the Human Stress Response." *PloS One* 8, no. 8 (August 2013): e70156, https://doi.org/10.1371/journal.pone.0070156.

According to the NorthShore: "9 Health Benefits of Music," NorthShore University HealthSystem, December 31, 2020, https://www.northshore.org /healthy-you/9-health-benefits-of-music.

Among the symposium participants: Emily Saarman, "Feeling the Beat: Symposium Explores the Therapeutic Effects of Rhythmic Music," *Stanford Report*, May 31, 2006, https://news.stanford.edu/news/2006/may31 /brainwave-053106.html.

"A lot of things": Jaime Alspach (music therapist), in discussion with the author, January 18, 2022.

Research reveals: Laura Ferreri et al., "Dopamine Modulates the Reward Experiences Elicited by Music," *Proceedings of the National Academy of Sciences* 116, no. 9 (January 2019): 3793–98, https://doi.org/10.1073 /pnas.1811878116.

Another study: Yuna L. Ferguson and Kennon M. Sheldon, "Trying to Be Happier Really Can Work: Two Experimental Studies," *Journal of Positive Psychology* 8, (2013): 23–33, https://doi.org/10.1080/17439760.2012.747000.

Making music: Rohit S. Loomba et al., "Effects of Music on Systolic Blood Pressure, Diastolic Blood Pressure, and Heart Rate: A Meta Analysis," *Indian Heart Journal* 64, no. 3 (May 2012): 309–13, https://doi.org/10.1016 /S0019-4832(12)60094-7.

And decrease your heart rate: Hans-Joachim Trappe and Gabriele Voit, "The Cardiovascular Effect of Muscial Genres," *Deutsches Arzteblatt International* 113, no. 20 (May 2016): 347–52, https://www.ncbi.nlm.nih.gov/pmc/articles /PMC4906829/.

"It's a good distraction": Ava Petlin (musician), in discussion with the author, February 10, 2022.

An article published: Ferris Jabr, "Let's Get Physical: The Psychology of Effective Workout Music," *Scientific American*, March 20, 2013, https://www .scientificamerican.com/article/psychology-workout-music/.

The London-based writer: Valentina Valentini (white noise enthusiast), in discussion with the author, January 14, 2022.

She isn't surprised: Dr. Jennifer Mundt (sleep psychologist), in discussion with the author, January 14, 2022.

This is why: J. R. Thorpe, "Here's What Happens in Your Brain When You Hear Noise," *Bustle*, November 6, 2019, https://www.bustle.com/p/what-white -noise-does-to-your-brain-according -to-experts-19271146.

When you breathe deeply: Jones, discussion.

According to the University of Rochester: Sara Smith, "5-4-3-2-1 Coping Technique for Anxiety," *Behavioral Health Partners* (blog), University of Rochester Medical Center, April 10, 2018, https://www.urmc.rochester .edu/behavioral-health-partners/bhp-blog/april-2018/5-4-3-2-1-coping -technique-for-anxiety.aspx.

"Though anxiety is": UR Medicine, "Hand on Heart Anxiety Reduction Technique," Youtube Video, 2:02, December 21, 2020, https://www.youtube. com/watch?v=2-WMJpoi8Qo.

A study referenced: B. Grace Bullock, "What Focusing on the Breath Does to Your Brain," *Greater Good Magazine*, October 31, 2019, https://greatergood.berkeley .edu/article/item/what_focusing_on_the_breath_does_to_your_brain.

"It's a way to connect": Christine Esposito (director and lead curator of Third Coast Disrupted: Artists + Scientists on Climate), in discussion with the author, March 2, 2022.

Bird watching, or birding: Jacey Fortin, "The Birds Are Not on Lockdown, and More People Are Watching Them," *New York Times*, May 29, 2020, https://www.nytimes.com/2020/05/29/science/bird-watching-coronavirus .html.

For those who suffer: Christopher W. Leahy, "Teaching Your Mind to Fly: The Psychological Benefits of Birdwatching," Princeton University Press, July 13, 2021, https://press.princeton.edu/ideas/teaching-your-mind-to-fly-the -psychological -benefits-of-birdwatching.

"It's quite meditative": Jacey Fortin, "The Birds Are Not on Lockdown, and More People Are Watching Them," *New York Times*, May 29, 2020, https:// www.nytimes.com/2020/05/29/science/bird-watching-coronavirus. html.

While watching birds: Daniel T. C. Cox et al., "Doses of Neighborhood Nature: The Benefits for Mental Health of Living with Nature," *BioScience* 67, no. 2 (February 2017): 147–55, https://doi.org/10.1093/biosci /biw173.

As Marta Curti reminds us: Marta Curti, "Ornitherapy: The Therapeutic Power of Birdwatching," *Birdwatching*, May 11, 2021, https://www.birdwatchingdaily .com/news/birdwatching/ornitherapy-therapeutic-power-birdwatching/.

According to Curti: Marta Curti, "Ornitherapy."

"These walks are": Christine Esposito (director and lead curator of Third Coast Disrupted: Artists + Scientists on Climate), in discussion with the author, March 2, 2022.

"Sound healing": Joanne Dusatko (sound healing and therapy practitioner), in discussion with the author, April 1, 2022.

One observational study: Tamara L. Goldsby et al., "Effects of Singing Bowl

Sound Meditation on Mood, Tension, and Well Being: An Observational Study," *Journal of Evidence-Based Complementary Alternative Medicine* 22, no. 3 (July 2017): 401–406, https://doi.org/10.1177/2156587216668109.

According to the study: Goldsby et al., "Effects of Singing Bowl."

What they learned: Goldsby et al., "Effects of Singing Bowl."

"You're standing": Barbara Senn (artist), in discussion with the author, March 29, 2022.

As of May 2022: "2021 Global Podcast Statistics, Demographics and Habits," PodcastHosting.org, April 19, 2021, https://podcasthosting.org/podcast-statistics.

More than half: "2021 Global Podcast Statistics."

One study published: Alexander G. Huth et al., "Natural Speech Reveals the Semantic Maps That Tile Human Cerebral Cortex," *Nature* 532 , (April 2016): 453–58, https://doi.org/10.1038/nature17637.

Some may experience: Huth et al., "Natural Speech."

While Seglin listens: Tracy Seglin (freelance writer and podcast enthusiast), in discussion with the author, May 20, 2022.

The reason might be: Hannah Malach, "How Listening to Podcasts Can Benefit Your Brain," *Good Housekeeping*, September 22, 2020, https://www.goodhousekeeping.com/health/wellness/a34100126/podcast-brain-benefits/.

"Your brain interprets": Malach, "How Listening to Podcasts."

Bunting also loves: Shannan Hofman Bunting (communications professional and podcast enthusiast), in discussion with the author, April 18, 2022.

SEE

"The question is": *Oxford Essential Quotations*, 5th ed., s.v. "Henry David Thoreau," accessed May 22, 2023, https://www.oxfordreference.com/display/10.1093/acref/9780191843730.001.0001/q-oro-ed5-00010905.

Indoor houseplants: Linjing Deng and Qihong Deng, "The Basic Roles of Indoor Plants in Human Health and Comfort," *Environmental Science and Pollution Research* 25, (November 2018): 36087–101, https://doi.org/10.1007/s11356-018-3554-1.

Since we spend: U.S. Environmental Protection Agency, *Report to Congress on Indoor Air Quality, vol. II, Assessment and Control of Indoor Air Pollution* (Washington, DC: EPA, 1989).

"Compared to previous years": Sierra Allen, "The Houseplant Hype," Nursery Management, April 2021, https://www.nurserymag.com/article/houseplant-hype-2021/.

According to Holli Schippers: Allen, "The Houseplant Hype."

Justin Hancock: Allen, "The Houseplant Hype."

"The only way to clean": Elvin McDonald, *Plants as Therapy* (New York: Praeger, 1976).

Results from a research study: Min-sun Lee et al., "Interaction with Indoor Plants May Reduce Psychological and Physiological Stress by Suppressing Autonomic Nervous System Activity in Young Adults: A Randomized Crossover Study," *Journal of Physiological Anthropology* 34, no. 1 (April 2015): 21, https://doi.org/10.1186/s40101-015-00 60-8.

"When you're on top": Elvin McDonald, *Plants as Therapy* (New York: Praeger Publishers, January 1976), 30-31.

"Grooming the right number": McDonald, Plants as Therapy, 35.

Some of us experience: "Shining a Light on Winter Depression," Harvard Health Publishing, November 1, 2019, https://www.health.harvard.edu/mind-and -mood/shining-a-light-on -winter-depression.

"SAD is not": "Shining a Light."

A prescription isn't necessary: "Seasonal Depression (Seasonal Affective Disorder)," Cleveland Clinic, April 10, 2022, https://my.clevelandclinic.org /health/diseases/9293-seasonal-depression.

"As days become longer": Harvard Health Publishing, "Shining a Light on Winter Depression," November 1, 2019, https://www.health.harvard.edu/ mind-and-mood/shining-a-light-on -winter-depression.

For SAD: "Seasonal Affective Disorder Treatment: Choosing a Light Box," Mayo Clinic, March 30, 2022, https://www.mayoclinic.org/tests-procedures /light-therapy/about/pac-20384604.

"Digital technology": John Miedema, "Slow Reading in an Information Ecology," in *Slow Reading* (Sacramento, CA: Litwin Books, 2009), https://litwinbooks .com/slow-reading/.

Lambert likens the idea: Ellen Lambert (former high school English teacher), in discussion with the author, February 16, 2022.

In his book: Miedema, *Slow Reading.*

"We cannot accelerate": Miedema, *Slow Reading.*

As we mature: Leatrice Eiseman (color specialist and executive director of the Pantone Color Institute), in discussion with the author, October 18, 2021.

Dr. Somia Gul notes: Somia Gull, Rabia Khalid Nadeem, and Anum Aslam, "Chromo Therapy—An Effective Treatment Option or Just a Myth?? Critical Analysis on the Effectiveness of Chromo Therapy," *American Research Journal of Pharmacy* 1, no. 2 (January 2015): 62–70, https://www.researchgate.net /publication/287196164_Chromo_therapy-_An_Effective_Treatment_Option _or_Just_a_Myth_Critical_Analysis_on_the_Effectiveness_of_Chromo_therapy.

While a fair amount: Andrew J. Elliot, "Color and Psychological Functioning: A Review of Theoretical and Empirical Work," *Frontiers in Psychology* 6, (April 2015): 368, https://doi.org/10.3389/fpsyg .2015.00368.

In a Q&A published: Dan Campbell, "This Is Your Brain on Art: A Q&A with Oshin Vartanian," *U of T News*, July 18, 2014, https://www.utoronto.ca/news /your- brain-art-q-oshin-vartanian.

According to Vartanian: Campbell, "This Is Your Brain on Art."

Phyl Terry isn't surprised: Phyl Terry (founder of Slow Art Day), in discussion with the author, May 6, 2022.

Maggie Levine is drawn: Maggie Levine (founder of Substack newsletter called ARTWRITE), in discussion with the author, April 6, 2022.

In a report published: Jocelyn Dodd and Ceri Jones, "Mind, Body, Spirit: How Museums Impact Health and Wellbeing," Research Centre for Museums and Galleries, School of Museum Studies, University of Leicester, June 2014, https://figshare.le.ac.uk/articles/report/Mind_Body_Spirit_How_museums _impact_health_and_wellbeing/10137716.

One of those programs: "Meetme, the MoMA's Alzheimer's Project: Making Art Accessible to People with Dementia," Museum of Modern Art 2022, http:// www.moma.org/meetme/.

Levine's Substack newsletter: Maggie Levine, "ARTWRITE,", accessed May 13, 2022 , https://artwrite.substack.com/.

"This is the genius": Christopher André, *Looking at Mindfulness: Twenty-Five Paintings to Change the Way You Live* (New York: Blue Rider Press, 2016), 2.

In 2016: Jordan Gaines Lewis, "A Neuroscientist Patiently Explains the Allure of the Adult Coloring Book," The Cut, January 10, 2016, https://www.thecut .com/2016/01/neuroscientist-explains-adult-coloring-books.html.

Nathalie Kunin doesn't: Nathalie Kunin (consultant and paint-by-numbers artist), in discussion with the author, May 2, 2022.

In a study: Nancy Curry and Tim Kasser, "Can Coloring Mandalas Reduce Anxiety?," *Art Therapy: Journal of the American Art Therapy Association* 22, no. 2 (2005): 81–85, https://files.eric.ed .gov/fulltext/EJ688443.pdf.

Johanna Basford, an illustrator: "Artist Goes Outside the Lines with Coloring Books for Grown-Ups," *NPR*, April 1, 2015, https://www.npr .org/2015/04/01/396634471/artist-goes-outside-the-lines-with-coloring -books-for-grown-ups.

According to some estimates: Jim Sollisch, "The Cure for Decision Fatigue," *Wall Street Journal*, June 10, 2016, https://www.wsj.com/articles /the-cure-for-decision-fatigue-1465596928.

According to Brandon Oto: Brandon Oto, "When Thinking Is Hard: Managing Decision Fatigue," *EMS World* 41, no. 5 (May 2012): 46–50, https:// www.hmpgloballearningnetwork.com/site/emsworld/article/10687160 /when-thinking-hard-managing-decision-fatigue.

In an effort: Christy Pino (one-hundred-day dress challenge participant), in discussion with the author, January 24, 2022.

Eby isn't surprised: Rebecca Eby (customer experience manager for Wool&), in discussion with the author, January 19, 2022.

In early 2021: Andrew Perrin and Sara Atske, "About Three-in-Ten U.S. Adults Say They Are 'Almost Constantly' Online," Pew Research Center, March 26, 2021, https://www.pewresearch.org/fact-tank/2021/03/26/about-three-in-ten -u-s-adults-say-they-are-almost-con stantly-online/.

Almost half: Perrin and Atske, "About Three-in-Ten."

In a piece: Brian X. Chen, "It's Time for a Digital Detox. (You Know You Need It.)," *New York Times*, November 25, 2020, https://www.nytimes.com/2020/11/25/technology/personaltech/digital-detox.html.

Round-the-clock monitoring: William J. Becker, Liuba Belkin, and Sarah Tuskey, "Killing Me Softly: Electronic Communications Monitoring and Employee and Spouse Well Being," *Academy of Management Proceedings* 2018, no. 1 (July 2018), https://doi.org/10.5465/AMBPP.2018.121.

Checking your email less overall: Kostadin Kushlev and Elizabeth W. Dunn, "Checking Email Less Frequently Reduces Stress," *Computers in Human Behavior* 43, (February 2015): 220–28, https://doi.org/10.1016/j.chb.2014.11.005.

In a study: Sara Thomée, "Mobile Phone Use and Mental Health: A Review of the Research That Takes a Psychological Perspective on Exposure," *International Journal of Environmental Research and Public Health* 15, no. 12 (November 2018): 2692, https://doi.org/10.3390/ijerph15122692.

While the study: Thomée, "Mobile Phone Use."

Before our digital devices: David J. Levitin, *The Organized Mind* (New York: Dutton, 2014), 171.

In one study: Darby E. Saxbe and Rena Repetti, "No Place Like Home: Home Tours Correlate with Daily Patterns of Mood and Cortisol," *Personality and Social Psychology Bulletin* 36, no. 1 (January 2010): 71–81, https://doi.org/10.1177/0146167209352864.

"We've evolved a preference": Alice Boyes, "6 Benefits of an Uncluttered Space," *Psychology Today*, February 12, 2018, https://www.psychologytoday.com/us/blog/in-practice/201802/6-benefits-uncluttered-space.

According to Regina Lark: Mary Macvean, "For Many People, Gathering Possessions Is Just the Stuff of Life," *Los Angeles Times*, March 21, 2014, https://www.latimes.com/health/la-xpm-2014-mar-21-la-he-keeping-stuff-20140322-story.html.

Part of the appeal: Marie Kondo, *The Life-Changing Magic of Tidying Up* (Berkeley, CA: Ten Speed Press, 2014).

"I would start": Jamie Gold (wellness design consultant and author), in discussion with the author, January 14, 2022.

Svetlana Battaglin once read: Svetlana Battaglin (amateur photographer), in discussion with the author, April 26, 2022.

A study published: "Daily Photography Improves Wellbeing: Taking a Photo Each Day and Posting It Online Has Complex Benefits," *ScienceDaily*, April 30, 2018, https://www.sciencedaily.com/releases/2018/04/180430131759.htm.

According to one participant: "Daily Photography."

Another participant: "Daily Photography."

"We show that": "Take a Picture, You'll Enjoy It More: Photographing Experiences Usually Increases Positive Feelings about Them, Study Says," *ScienceDaily*, June 9, 2016, https://www.sciencedaily.com/releases/2016/06/160609174804.htm.

"One critical factor": "Take a Picture."

"We really do try": Christina Schleich (lead organizer of the Avondale Gardening Association), in discussion with the author, May 24, 2022.

While it's not unique: "Neighborhood, Not Metaverse: Venn's 2021 Trends Report," Venn, 2022, https://global.venn.city/neighborhood-trends-report-2021/.

Mental Health America found: "How Connections Help," Mental Health America, 2022, https://www.mhanational.org/connect-others.

While most people know: "The Science of Kindness," Cedars Sinai, February 13, 2019, https://www.cedars-sinai.org/blog/science-of-kindness.html.

In another report: Debra Umberson and Jennifer Karas Montez, "Social Relationships and Health: A Flashpoint for Health Policy," *Journal of Health and Social Behavior* 51, Supplement (2010): S54–66, https://doi.org/10.1177/0022146510383501.

According to the *Harvard Women's Health Watch*: "The Health Benefits of Strong Relationships," *Harvard Women's Health Watch*, December 1, 2010, https://www.health.harvard.edu/staying-healthy/the-health-benefits-of-strong-relationships.

"Dozens of studies": "Health Benefits."

According to the report: "Health Benefits."

According to IsHak: "Science of Kindness."

"The rewards of acts of kindness": "Science of Kindness."

Grounding, she says: Olga Mecking (writer), in discussion with the author, May 20, 2022.

"Downtime is more about": David Rock et al., "The Healthy Mind Platter," *NeuroLeadership Journal* 4, (October 2012): 8, https://davidrock.net/files/02_The_Healthy_Mind_Platter_US.pdf.

In her TED Talk in 2017: Manoush Zomorodi, "How Boredom Can Lead to Your Most Brilliant Ideas," filmed April 27, 2017, in Vancouver, BC, TED video, 15:34, https://www.ted.com/talks/manoush_zomorodi_how_boredom_can_lead_to_your_most_brilliant_ideas.

The University of Virginia psychologist: Wilson et al., "Just Think."

"In many ways": David Rock et al., "The Healthy Mind Platter," *NeuroLeadership Journal*, NeuroLeadership Journal 4 (October 2012): 8.

As Mecking reminds readers: Olga Mecking, *Niksen: Embracing the Dutch Art of Doing Nothing* (Boston: Houghton Mifflin Harcourt, 2020), 165.

INDEX

ABOUT THE AUTHOR

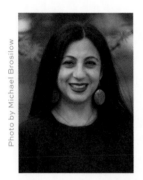

Megy Karydes is a Chicago-based writer and communications professional. Her work has appeared in *USA Today, National Geographic, The Atlantic, Sierra Club, Forbes, Eating Well, Architectural Digest, Midwest Living*, and elsewhere. Megy also helped lead and manage communications campaigns and projects for science-focused and social justice organizations. She teaches graduate-level communications courses at Johns Hopkins University. She journals every morning and does kickboxing at night as a way to de-stress after a long day. She lives with her husband, two teenagers, and their dog who barks indiscriminately at all outdoor decorations, whether it's Halloween décor or Baby Jesus in a manger during her daily walks. When she's not lost in a good book or trying a new indie restaurant in town, you can find her at MegyKarydes.com.